When
Your
Child
Struggles

When Your Child Struggles

The Myths of 20/20 Vision
What Every Parent Needs to Know

David L. Cook, O.D.

Invision Press, Atlanta

Copyright © 2004 David L. Cook
Second Edition
Printed in the United States of America

Library of Congress Catalog Card Number:
92-071000
ISBN 0-9632657-0-9

Published by Invision Press, Atlanta, Georgia

Author Contact Information

If you have questions or comments, Dr. Cook would enjoy hearing from you.

E-mail: cook2020@aol.com

Mail: Dr. David L. Cook
Cook Vision Therapy Center, Inc.
1395 S. Marietta Parkway
Building 400, Suite 107
Marietta, Georgia 30067

Phone: Local (770) 419-0400

For more information on vision therapy for adults read *VISUAL FITNESS: 7 Minutes to Better Eyesight and Beyond*, or visit www.cookvisiontherapy.com.

Also by David Cook, O.D.

VISION:
What Every Pilot Needs to Know

VISUAL FITNESS:
7 Minutes to Better Eyesight and Beyond

*To the thousands of parents who have shared
this book with others searching for answers—
My heartfelt thanks*

The eye movement test in Chapter 8 is directly based on the K-D Test, available from Bernell Corporation, 750 Lincolnway East, P.O. Box 4637, South Bend, Indiana 46634. The publisher would also like to thank them for granting permission to use their acuity figures shown on page 31.

Acknowledgments

I'd like to thank the following experts on developmental vision and vision therapy for their insights and support (by state):

Alaska:

Dr. Jeffrey G. Keene
16331 Heritage Place, Ste. 103
Eagle River, AK 99577
(907) 694-4420
vtc@gci.net

California:

Dr. Beth Ballinger
Dr. Steven Cohn
901 Dover Drive, Ste. 100
Newport Beach, CA 92660
fourvision@yahoo.com

Dr. Penelope S. Suter
5300 Lennox Avenue, Ste. 101
Bakersfield, CA 93309
(661) 869-2010
drsuter101@ hotmail.com

Massachusetts

Dr. John M. Abbondanza
30 Turnpike Rd. ,Ste. 7
Southborough, MA 01772
(508) 481-8558
dr.john@greatvisioncare.com

Dr. Cathy Stern
7 Cedar Drive
Canton, MA 02021
(781) 575-0057
www.myvisiondoc.com

Michigan

Dr. Dan L. Fortenbacher
2908 Division Street
St. Joseph, MI 49085
(616) 983-3309
wow@wowvision.net

New Jersey

Dr. Nickolas Despotidis
Dr. Barry M. Tannen
1777 Kuser Road
Hamilton Square, NJ 08690
(609) 581-5755
btannenod@aol.com

Dr. Leonard Press
17-10 Fair Lawn Ave., 2nd Floor
Fair Lawn, NJ 07410
(201) 794-7977
pressvision@aol.com

Nebraska

Dr. Vicky Vandervort
Dr. Will Ferguson
9900 Nicholas St. Ste 250
Omaha, NE 68114
(402) 493-6500
www.Heartland-Eye.com

New York

Dr. Samantha Slotnick
161 S Central Park Ave.
Hartsdale, NY 10530
(914) 874-1118
www.Dr Slotnick.com

Dr. Gary J. Williams
Dr. Stephen S. Solomon
293 Main Street
Owego, NY 13827
(607) 687-3391

Oregon

Dr. Gabby Marshall
Elemental Eyecare
2736 NW Crossing Dr., Ste 120
Bend, OR 97701
(541) 323-3937
www.elementaleyecare.com

Texas

Dr. Desiree Hopping
1234 Bay Area Blvd., Ste. E
Houston, TX 77058
(281) 488-2020
DTHopping@aol.com

Dr. Briana M Larson
10601 Pecan Park Blvd., #201
Austin, TX 78750
(512) 401-0400
www.ocvt.info

Dr. Emily Schottman
Dr. Mary McMains
2116 Austin, TX 78756
(512) 419-1212
www.austinvt .com

Utah

Dr. Robin Price
908 N. 2000 W.
Pleasant Grove, UT 84062
(801) 492-6393
drprice@utahvisioncare.com

Virginia

Dr. Tod R. Davis
7001 Heritage Dr. # 175
Gainesville, VA 20155-3151
(703) 753- 9777
www.davisvisiontherapy.com

Washington

Dr. Todd Wylie
412 East 30th Avenue
Spokane, WA 99203
(509) 535-5855
dtw@cet.com

Washington (cont.)

Dr. Nancy Torgerson
16006 Ash Way # 101
Lynnwood, WA 98087
(425) 787-5200
nancyt@nwlink.com

West Virginia

Dr. Gary G. Veronneau
1102 Main Street
Rainelle, WV 25962
(304) 438-8574
ldoc@citynet.net

Wisconsin

Dr. Ann Wonderling
3424 Mormon Coulee Road,
Ste. B
LaCrosse, WI 54601
(608) 788-5380
www.visiontherapyacademy.com

Dr. Richard Foss
3424 Mormon Coulee Road
Ste. B
LaCrosse, WI 54601
(608) 788-4300
www.wifamilyvisioncenter.com

Alberta, Canada

Dr. Brent Neufeld
2880 GlenmoreTrail SE, Ste. 130
Calgary, AB, Canada, T2C 2E7
(403) 242-1800
drneufeld@calgaryvision
therapy.com

Contents

Introduction

Why write a book for parents about their children's vision?

Oddly enough, much of the momentum I needed to make time for writing came from my work with adults rather than children. Over the past several years I have seen a growing number of adults with vision problems which were previously undiscovered because these adults could easily read the smallest letters on an eye chart.

Most of these adults who were motivated enough to come to us to handle these vision problems had, before they reached us, already succeeded in their careers. The majority were in business for themselves.

While these adults came from many different lines of work, they all had one thing in common: their undetected vision problems had caused them to endure the humiliation of having difficulty learning to read. As a result, despite an outward appearance of confidence and success, they secretly felt stupid because they had experienced such a struggle with reading.

For some, the struggle had been so great that as I told them that there was hope, they cried. One gentleman went so far as to tell me, "I feel as if I've wasted 16 years!"

The sad thing is that his "waste" was unnecessary. He could have been helped when he was a child. But why wasn't he? Why do such children have to go through school feeling frustrated and stupid and losing self-esteem?

The answer, as we will see in this book, is not exactly simple, but it rests on the following fact: parents have not been taught what to look for and don't know where to find help.

As I continue to see adults who have suffered from undetected vision problems and hear their stories of frustration, humiliation, or anger, I become more and more resolved to see that parents receive the information they need to end their children's unnecessary struggles.

It is to help end these struggles that this book was written.

SECTION 1
Understanding 20/20

CHAPTER 1

The Most Dangerous Assumption

T he word "assumption" can be defined as "anything that you SUPPOSE to be a fact." With this definition in mind we can ask a question which may—whether you know it or not—be seriously affecting your child's life:

WHAT IS THE MOST DANGEROUS ASSUMPTION THAT YOU, AS A PARENT, CAN MAKE ABOUT YOUR CHILD'S VISION?

Before answering this question, let us look at some information.

First, this "dangerous assumption" is all too common. Some parents make it after their child has passed a school vision screening. Other parents make this assumption after the eye test in the pediatrician's office reveals no problem. Still other parents make this assumption after a trip to the eye doctor has shown the child to have healthy eyes and the ability to read the tiniest letters on a chart at the end of a long room.

It is true that in three out of four cases the assumption is correct and, therefore, causes no problems. Perhaps this is why the assumption is so common.

It is equally true that in one case in four the assumption is false and results in an unhappy child who struggles while you stand by feeling hopeless or sad or frustrated or angry about your child's inablility to succeed—despite BOTH of your best efforts.

In almost a decade and a half of practice, I've witnessed parents from all walks of life make the wrong assumption, through no fault of their own. Homemakers, carpenters, educators, and especially doctors—all have made the assumption and all have watched as their children failed to reach desired goals.

Have you yourself made this "dangerous assumption?" If so, your child may already be falling into one of several patterns of behavior. The following ten questions will give you a clue if such is the case:

1. Is your child struggling and frustrated in school even though you know he or she is bright?

2. Does homework, which should take minutes in

stead of hours, drag on all evening and sometimes end up with you losing your patience or your child becoming frustrated or even crying?

3. Do you have a child who does not read for fun and may NEVER develop a love of reading?

4. Is your child struggling to learn to read, dropping out small words and filling in words that aren't really there, failing to recognize the same word in a later line which you taught him on an earlier line?

5. Is it difficult for your child to complete any writing or boardwork or to get his thoughts down on paper even though he or she is highly verbal and can easily answer your questions at home and the teacher's questions in class?

6. Does your child struggle to learn spelling words for the test and then forget them as soon as the test is over?

7. Do you have a child who learned how to read easily in first, second, and third grade, but beginning in fourth grade began to have difficulty with reading subjects such as reading, social studies, and science?

8. Is your child a better reader on the first page than after reading several pages? Does he or she start out fine and then begin to squirm or want to get away?

9. Does your child recognize the words when reading but still have trouble with reading comprehension?

10. Is your child's frustration in school causing him to be labelled as being somehow "disabled" or a "behavior problem" or having an "attention deficit" even though you are not aware of these problems at home, except when schoolwork is mentioned?

Each of the behaviors listed in these ten questions can be related to a different vision problem, which when overlooked, may cause your child, and you, to suffer.

If you answered "yes" to ANY of these questions, then you have a real and legitimate cause for concern or upset. If this upset has gone on long enough it may even be making it difficult for you to enjoy the time you spend with your child.

The real question is, however, how will these problems be affecting you and your child five years from now? When you consider this last question, it may seem to you that it's time for things to improve.

Fortunately, despite the seriousness of this subject, there is some good news: a solution exists, and information on that solution is contained in this book.

The following is the PURPOSE of this book:

TO ALLOW PARENTS TO UNDERSTAND VISION WELL ENOUGH TO KNOW WHEN AND WHERE TO FIND HELP FOR THEIR CHILDREN.

Upon completing this book, you, as a parent, should have gained the following two abilities:

1. TO UNDERSTAND VISION THOROUGHLY ENOUGH TO ALLOW YOU TO SPOT THE VISION PROBLEMS WHICH MIGHT OTHERWISE REDUCE YOUR CHILD'S SUCCESS.

2. TO KNOW WHERE TO TURN FOR AID WHEN THE SCHOOL SCREENING OR A TRIP TO THE DOCTOR'S OFFICE DO NOT EXPLAIN HOW TO HELP YOUR CHILD.

To help you gain these two abilities, this book is divided into three sections. Section I will give you the ability to understand the information which can be obtained through a school screening or routine eye examination. Section II will allow you to understand visual conditions which are frequently overlooked during screenings and routine eye examinations. Section III will inform you on what help is available and how to find that help.

If your child is struggling, this book is for you. In the chapters which follow, you will learn more about the "dangerous assumption" and the way that assumption may be affecting your child's life.

CHAPTER 2

The Battle Against
Poor Eyesight

Т**he Battle Begins**

In 1862, during the time of the Civil War, a man by the name of Snellen started a battle of a different kind—a battle against poor eyesight. Snellen started this battle by inventing a chart for testing eyes.

Snellen's chart consisted of letters of different sizes. Individuals were asked to stand twenty feet away from the chart and read its letters. Those who could read the letters were assumed to have won the battle against poor eyesight. Those who could not read the letters were assumed to have lost.

Today, over a century and a quarter later, when your child's eyesight is tested, the "weapons," or rather the instruments used to perform the exam, are far more advanced than those of the last century, but the battle is pretty much the same. The child who reads the chart wins; the child who fails to read the chart loses.

Snellen's chart is a means of measuring one ability of your child to see: *visual acuity*.

Visual Acuity Defined

Visual acuity is the term we use to describe "sharpness of sight" especially the ability to discern small details. The word *acuity* comes from the Latin *acutus* meaning sharp.

Your child's ability to see small letters across the room is an example of good visual acuity. Without such an ability, a child sitting in the back of the classroom would not be able to see the chalkboard.

Measuring Visual Acuity

When measuring the visual acuity of a child who already knows the alphabet, we will normally show the child letters of gradually decreasing size at approximately a twenty foot distance. We will begin with letters that your child can easily read and then continue on to smaller and smaller letters until your child can no longer identify them.

When this testing is complete, we write down the results using a fraction which contains two numbers.

The top number of the fraction represents the distance at which your child identified the letters. The fraction's bottom number represents the size of the smallest letters seen. We call this fraction a *Snellen Fraction.*

Possibly the best known Snellen fraction is 20/20. The first 20 tells us that the test was performed at the commonly used 20-foot testing distance which Snellen himself suggested.

The second 20 in the fraction refers to the size of the smallest letters seen. This 20 stands for the smallest letter size that a person with supposedly "normal" acuity can see when standing twenty feet away from the letter. We, therefore, consider 20/20 to be "normal" visual acuity.

We expect many kindergarten children and most first-graders to be able to read the 20/20 letters. The letters in Figure 1 are examples of 20/20 letters. If you and your child can see these letters at 20 feet, then you and your child have 20/20 acuity.

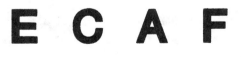

Figure 1

In the Snellen fraction 20/25, the 20 again stands for the 20-foot examination distance. The 25 stands for the size of letter that a person with normal acuity should be able to see at 25 feet. The letters in Figure 2 are examples of 20/25 letters. The child with 20/25 acuity obviously cannot see smaller letters as well as a child with 20/20.

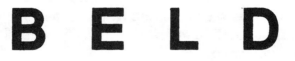

25-Foot Letters

Figure 2

The next larger letters are 20/30 letters. The smallest letters that a child with 20/30 acuity is able to identify are the same letters that a person with normal acuity can see at 30 feet. Examples of 20/30 letters are found in Figure 3.

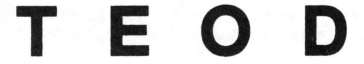

30-Foot Letters

Figure 3

The 20/40 letters (Figure 4) are the next larger letters which appear on a chart for measuring acuity. These letters are twice as large as the 20/20 letters. If these are the smallest letters that your child can read at 20 feet, then your child's acuity is 20/40.

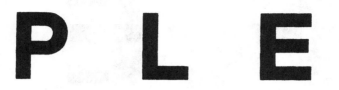

40-Foot Letters

Figure 4

The next larger letters on the acuity chart are the 20/50 letters (see Figure 5). If these are the smallest letters that your child can read at 20 feet, then your child's acuity is 20/50.

50-Foot Letters

Figure 5

Larger than the 20/50 letters are the 20/60 letters (Figure 6), the 20/70 letters (Figure 7), the 20/80 letters (Figure 8), the 20/100 letters (Figure 9) and the 20/200 letter (Figure 10).

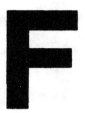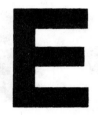

60-Foot Letters

Figure 6

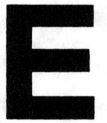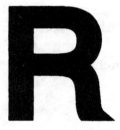

70-Foot Letters

Figure 7

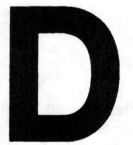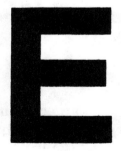

80-Foot Letters

Figure 8

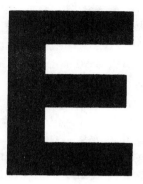

100-Foot Letters

Figure 9

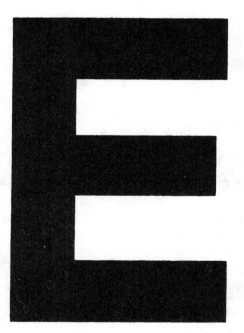

200-Foot Letters

Figure 10

The 20/60 letters are three times the size of the 20/20 letters, the 20/80 letters are four times the size of the 20/20 letters, the 20/100 letters are five times the size of the 20/20 letters, and the 20/200 letters are ten times the size of the 20/20 letters.

Even though 20/20 is considered "Normal Acuity," it is not perfect acuity. There exist acuity letters which are smaller than the 20/20 letters. The 20/15 letters are an example (Figure 11). A child with normal acuity has to move up to 15 feet to see these letters. A child with 20/15 acuity can see these letters at 20 feet.

L E F O D T

15-Foot Letters

Figure 11

Testing Younger Children

If your child has not yet thoroughly learned his alphabet, the examiner may use "E's" instead and ask your child to "point" the same way that the E's are pointing. For instance, in Figure 12, the E's point right, down, left and up.

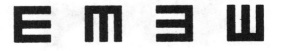

Figure 12

Another method we use to measure a young child's acuity is to show the child "pictures" rather than letters. An example of these "pictures" appears in Figure 13.

Figure 13

We begin with these pictures by asking your child to name them while they are positioned 10 to 16 inches away. If the names of the pictures are not known, we practice until your child can consistantly name the "birthday cake, hand, bird and horse."

Once your child can easily name the pictures within arm's reach, we show the pictures across the room. At this twenty foot distance, we begin with big pictures to build confidence. We then gradually move to the smallest pictures that your child can see.

Most three-year-olds already know, or can be taught to read, these pictures. For this reason, among others, age three is generally a convenient, and wise, time for a child's first exam (an earlier exam is, of course, recommended if you suspect any problem). We will say more about the need to have your child's eyes examined.

Reasons for Reduced Acuity

By *reduced acuity* we mean that a child's visual acuity is worse than 20/20 in one or both eyes. While there are many reasons why a child might have less than 20/20 acuity in an eye, the following are the major ones.

Immaturity

The most common reason why children under age six have reduced acuity is that their ability to understand what they see is too immature for them to recognize the letters or pictures used. If such immaturity continues past age five, your child may have a difficulty which could affect learning to read. This difficulty will be explained in Chapter 9.

Glasses

The most common reason why a child who is older than age six has reduced acuity is that glasses are needed. While wearing glasses, such children will again demonstrate normal acuity. The three main reasons why glasses may be necessary to restore acuity will be covered in Chapter 4.

Amblyopia

Approximately two or three children in every hundred have reduced vision for a more serious reason. They have Amblyopia. *Amblyopia* (also called *Lazy*

Eye) is a condition in which an eye does not learn to see correctly because that eye was "crossed" or because needed glasses were not obtained at an early enough age. When amblyopia is present, the vision in your child's lazy eye will remain reduced even when the "best" pair of glasses are worn.

Because amblyopia is usually present in only one eye, a child will frequently learn to depend on his better eye and show absolutely no signs of the condition that a parent can detect. This is another reason why we suggest that all children receive their first exam by age 3.

The most common myths about amblyopia and crossed-eyes as well as information about their treatment will be covered in Chapter 12 and Appendix A.

Eye Health

By far the least common reason for reduced acuity in children is eye health. In considering all persons under the age of 45, amblyopia—which is relatively infrequent itself—is responsible for more lost vision than ALL eye-health problems and eye accidents combined.

Even though lost acuity from eye-health problems is rare, all *optometrists* (see the glossary for the definition of "optometrist") carefully consider this area during a child's routine eye examination. As a parent, the best thing you can do to ensure that your child's eyes remain healthy is to have your child seen for yearly examinations.

Summary

In this chapter we have considered one visual ability: the ability of your child to see tiny details in the distance.

This ability, which is necessary to see the blackboard in school, is measured using a technique which was developed by Snellen in 1862. During many school vision screenings, and fortunately in a decreasing number of eye doctor's offices, the battle against poor eyesight is still being fought in much the same way it was fought during the Civil War. If your child sees 20/20, he wins. If he cannot see 20/20, he loses and gets glasses.

Unfortunately, the child with 20/20 acuity may all too often win the battle only to lose the war. Just what is meant by this statement will become apparent as, in future chapters, we provide additional information about the "most dangerous assumption" that you can make about your child's vision.

Drill

To check your child's visual acuity, while at the same time gaining a better understanding of the material in this chapter, perform the following drill.

Using the letters in Figures 1 through 10, find the smallest letters which you can see at 20 feet. Do this drill one eye at a time. For each eye, write down the smallest letters you were able to see at the 20 foot distance.

If, for instance, you can see the 20/20 letters with your right eye and the 20/30 letters with your left eye you would write down your acuity as follows: Right eye, 20/20; Left eye, 20/30.

When you have finished with your own eyes so that you are comfortable with the test, repeat the procedure with your child. Again, write down what you find*.

---

*The acuity letter sizes in this book, while very close to the standard letters found in a doctor's office, are approximate only. Acuity will also vary according to how much light is falling on the letters. Neither this drill, nor any of the drills which follow are a substitute for a complete eye-health evaluation with your family optometrist.

Chapter 3

Your Child's Eyes

Before you can understand how your child's eyes work, it is necessary to have some idea of the structure of those eyes. The following description is brief and includes only those details which you will need in later chapters to understand material which concerns your child.

The Eye

The eye is round like a ball. All we can see is the front surface of the eye (Figure 1). The rest of the eye is

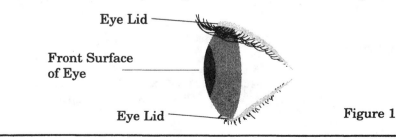

Eye Lid

Front Surface of Eye

Eye Lid

Figure 1

hidden behind the eyelids. Figure 2 is a top view of the entire eye, not just the part that can be seen between the eyelids. The figure is drawn as if you are looking at the eye from above and the top half of the eye has been removed to reveal the inside. The parts of the eye are labeled. A brief description of these parts will help you to understand later material in this book which may relate to your child. As you read about each part, you should find it on Figure 2.

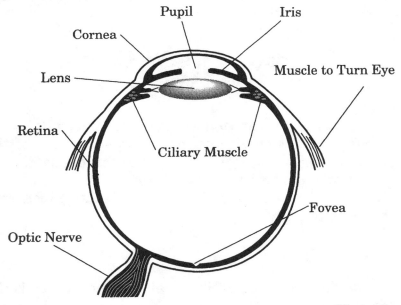

Figure 2

Cornea

The *cornea* is the transparent front surface of the eye. Light passes through the cornea into the eye.

When contact lenses are worn, they rest on the tears which cover the cornea.

Iris

The *iris* is located directly behind the cornea. It is the colored part of the eye. A person with "blue" eyes has blue irises.

Pupil

The *pupil* is the round dark opening in the center of the iris. This opening controls how much light enters the back of the eye. In the sunlight, the pupil constricts so as to help protect the rear of the eye from too much light. In the dark, the pupil expands to allow more light to reach the rear of the eye. Some children have very large pupils, others have small pupils. Such variation in pupil size is generally normal.

Lens

Behind the pupil is the *lens*. The lens is made out of flexible material and can change shape. The lens focuses light much as a magnifying glass does.

Ciliary Muscle

The *ciliary muscle* controls the shape of the lens. By making the lens more or less curved, the ciliary muscle allows the eye to be focused for seeing at different distances. The importance of this process will be further explained in Chapter 6 which concerns your child's ability to keep reading material clear.

Retina

The *retina* is like a movie screen on the back of the eye. This screen is made up of receptor cells which, when struck by light, send tiny electrical impulses to the brain via the *optic nerve*. When your child interprets the information reaching the brain, seeing occurs. In Chapters 9 through 11, we will say more about your child's ability to interpret and remember what is seen.

Fovea

The *fovea* is the area of the retina which has the greatest number of receptor cells. There are over a million receptor cells in this tiny central area of the retina. The further away from the fovea one travels in the retina, the fewer receptor cells there are. This is the reason why our central vision is better than peripheral vision. Why this information is important will become obvious when we discuss why children lose their place when reading in Chapter 8.

Muscles to Turn the Eye

The eye is moved by the muscles which surround it. There are six muscles around each eye (only two are shown in Figure 2). All twelve muscles must be perfectly coordinated for the two eyes to move together as a team rather than to "fight" one another. Again, this in formation will form the basis of Chapter 7 which relates to double vision and reading difficulty.

Drill

As a quick review of this chapter, provide the labels for the following diagram. Check yourself against Figure 2. The names of the parts of the eye will be used again in the chapters which follow.

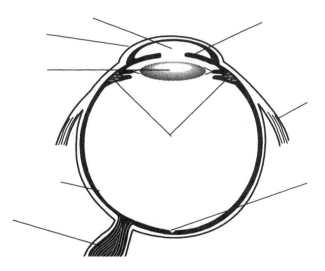

CHAPTER 4

Glasses—
Friend or Foe?

When do glasses help? When do they not help? There are times when glasses allow children to perform dramatically better in school. There are other instances when glasses provide parents with a false sense of security even when all is not yet well.

For this reason, every parent needs to be able to distinguish between these two conditions. In this chapter we are going to concentrate on your understanding of how glasses help. In later chapters we will provide information that will make it easier for you to spot when glasses are not doing the job.

Al's Story

Al was in fifth grade. He had a bad habit of sitting too close to the television set. A habit which, not infrequently, upset his father and led to arguments.

In school, Al was having difficulty finishing his boardwork. He was an excellent reader, however, and spent many hours each day reading for pleasure.

Finally, during the yearly school screening, it was discovered that Al's acuity was 20/200 in each eye. The 20/200 letters are twice the size of the 20/100 letters shown in Chapter 2. The family optometrist found that Al needed glasses to see far away.

When Al got home with his new glasses, he looked down the street and saw his uncle's house, a house he had walked to countless times in the past. All excited he exclaimed to his parents, "I didn't know you could see Uncle Ed's house from here!"

Al was lucky. His acuity was obviously worse than 20/20, so his seeing problem was detected on the school screening. Not every child who needs glasses is so lucky. There are children who need glasses even though they have 20/20 vision. Such children are not picked up on school screenings and can only be detected during a routine eye examination.

Before we can understand why the 20/20 screening misses certain problems which require glasses, we need to review some information which explains why glasses are prescribed.

To accomplish this end, we will begin with some necessary basics and then cover the three reasons for glasses.

Definition of Light

Light is a form of energy which, when it strikes the *retina* of the eye, causes the movement of signals from the eye to the brain. The interpretation of these signals results in vision (Figure 1).

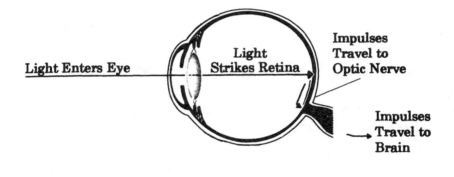

Figure 1

How Light Travels

Light travels along straight lines called rays. If the rays of light are gradually moving further apart, they are said to be *diverging*. If the rays are moving closer together, they are said to be *converging*. If the rays are traveling in the identical direction, they are said to be *parallel*. (See Figure 2).

45

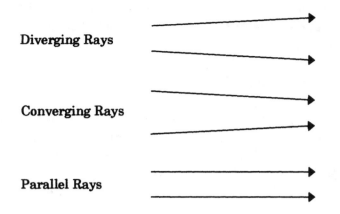

Figure 2

Lenses

A *lens* is transparent material which has at least one curved surface.

A *convex lens* is curved like the outside of a ball. It is thicker in the center than at the edges and causes light to converge (Figure 3). A magnifying glass is an

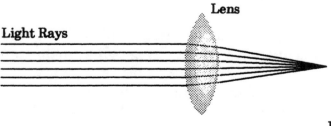

Figure 3

example of a convex lens. The *lens* of the eye (see Chapter 3) is another example of a convex lens.

A *concave lens* is curved like the inside of a ball. It is thicker on the edges than the center and causes light to diverge (Figure 4).

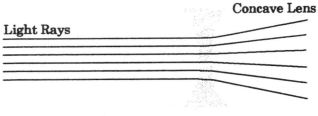

Figure 4

Focus of a Lens

The *focus* of a lens is the point where rays of light passing through the lens appear to meet (Figure 5). For instance, if we were trying to burn a hole in a leaf with a magnifying glass (convex lens), we would move the lens closer and further from the leaf until we got the focus of the lens right on the leaf.

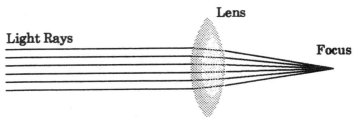

Figure 5

Power of a Lens

The stronger a lens is the more it will bend light and the closer the focus of the lens will be to the lens itself. The strength of a lens depends on its curvature. The more curved the lens, the stronger it is, and the less curved, the weaker (Figure 6).

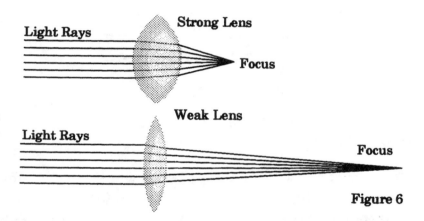

Figure 6

Where Light Comes From

A *light source*—that object such as the sun or a light bulb creating the light—gives off rays of light in all directions (Figure 7). When these light rays strike an

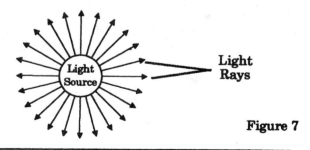

Figure 7

object they bounce off that object just like a billiard ball would bounce off the cushion of a pool table (Figure 8). The reason we are able to see objects is because the light which is reflected off these objects reaches our eyes.

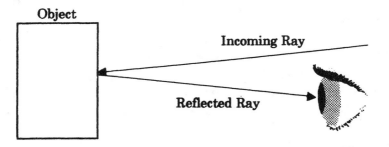

Object

Incoming Ray

Reflected Ray

Figure 8

Normal Eyes

When eyes are "normal" and do not require glasses for seeing in the distance, light coming from an acuity chart which is 20 feet away will enter the eyes through the pupils and be focused on the retina of each eye (Figure 9). This accurate focus will occur when the *ciliary muscles* (see Chapter 3) which control the shape

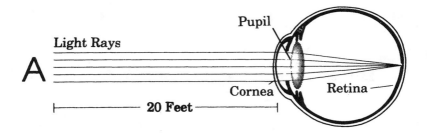

Light Rays

A

Pupil

Cornea

Retina

20 Feet

Figure 9

of the *lenses* of the eyes, are completely relaxed.

Thus when a child with "normal" eyes looks across the room at the chalkboard, the light coming from the board will be accurately focused on that child's retinas without the child having to work to contract his ciliary muscles to see.

In actual fact, not all children have "normal" eyes. There are three different vision problems which may require a child to wear glasses to see comfortably and clearly when looking at the chalkboard.

Myopia

Myopia is a kind of vision problem which makes it difficult to see far away without glasses or contact lenses. The popular term used to describe this condition is *nearsightedness*.

When a child has myopia, light coming from the chalkboard will be focused in front of the child's retinas (Figure 10). As a result, the child will struggle to see the chalkboard and likely fail the school vision screening.

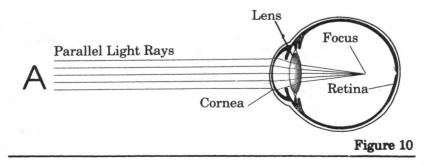

Figure 10

If the condition is mild, the child may be able to see the chalkboard when sitting in the front row. If the child is very nearsighted, things may be blurry even at arm's length. If this is the case, the child will probably hold reading material closer than expected so the words will remain clear. For this reason, nearsightedness usually does not affect reading. In fact, on the average, nearsighted children are better readers than farsighted children.

To compensate for the difficulty with distance seeing, concave lenses are prescribed for nearsightedness. These lenses cause the light to diverge enough to be focused on the retina (Figure 11). When wearing such glasses, the nearsighted child will, in most cases, again be able to see clearly in the distance.

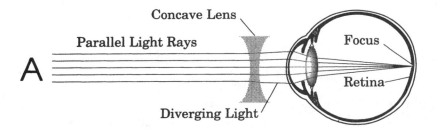

Figure 11

Hyperopia

Hyperopia is a condition in which light coming from the chalkboard is focused behind a child's retinas when the ciliary muscles are relaxed (Figure 12).

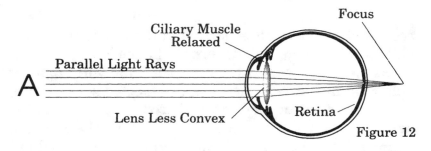

Figure 12

To see in the distance, the hyperopic child has to increase the power of the lenses inside his eyes. To do this, the child must tighten the ciliary muscles inside the eyes. This action results in the eyes' lenses increasing in curvature (Figure 13).

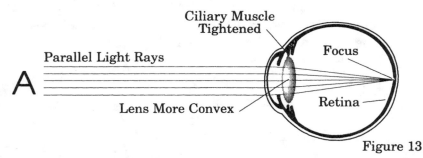

Figure 13

As explained in the "Power of the Lens" section above, the increase in curvature results in the light being focused closer to the lens. When this process is accurate, the light is focused on the retinas and vision is once again clear.

Unlike the nearsighted child who sees better up close than far away, the hyperopic child has more difficulty the closer he looks. For this reason, the popular term for hyperopia is *farsightedness*.

If talking to a farsighted child during an examination reveals that there are any symptoms of sore eyes, headaches, avoidance of reading, or difficulty in school, the optometrist is likely to prescribe *convex lenses*. These lenses focus the light on the retinas without the hyperopic child having to strain to tighten his ciliary muscles (Figure 14). The result can be a more comfortable and efficient child in school.

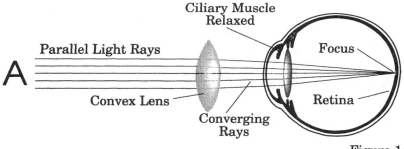

Figure 14

Because the hyperopic child is at times capable of tightening his ciliary muscles long enough to read an acuity chart, school vision screenings may fail to detect hyperopia. As a result, there are many children who pass the school screening only to continue to suffer from blurred vision during reading and boardwork.

Because hyperopia freqently goes undetected on school vision screenings, every child should have a thorough vision examination by the family optometrist to rule out this condition.

Astigmatism

Astigmatism is a condition in which the light rays entering the eye do not all converge to meet at the same focus. Instead, the rays meet at various distances in front of or behind the retina (Figure 15). As a result, the light which falls on the retina is distorted no matter what distance the child is looking. The term astigmatism is derived from the Greek words which roughly mean "without a point."

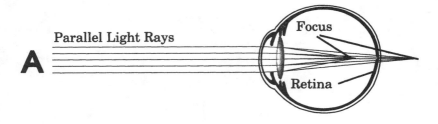

Figure 15

The child with astigmatism may have blurred vision both when looking at the chalkboard and when reading. Because of the way the light is distorted, children may be able to make out letters for the few seconds it takes to read the acuity chart even though vision is blurred at other times. Thus, some children who have enough astigmatism to require glasses may, nonetheless, pass the school vision screening.

Children who have astigmatism which is not corrected with glasses are likely to suffer from burning, uncomfortable eyes when reading and doing boardwork. Glasses can relieve these symptoms.

As with hyperopia, a complete eye examination is necessary to rule out the presence of astigmatism.

Summary

In this chapter we have covered the three reasons why glasses are prescribed for distance seeing: myopia, hyperopia, and astigmatism. When glasses are correctly prescribed for these conditions, visual acuity should in most cases be 20/20 when the glasses are worn. As mentioned above, even children who pass the school screening may still require glasses for comfortable and efficient seeing. For this reason, any child who is not doing as well in school as you would expect should have an examination.

Unfortunately, there are children who have 20/20 vision while wearing glasses or who require no glasses at all to see 20/20, who nonetheless suffer from other visual problems which make schoolwork difficult. Because a general eye exam is not designed to pick up these other problems, there are many children who have 20/20 vision and "normal eye exams" who still do not have the other visual abilities needed to succeed at school.

The "most dangerous assumption" which a parent can make regarding a child's vision is related to these vision problems which exist even in the presence of 20/20 acuity. This assumption will be clearly stated in the next chapter.

SECTION 2
The Visual Abilities

CHAPTER 5

The Dangers of
20/20 Eyesight

As we have covered in the preceding chapters, 20/20 acuity is the ability to see tiny letters in the distance. Some children need glasses to see 20/20. Others can see 20/20 without glasses. Obviously, 20/20 must be an asset. How, then, can 20/20 also be dangerous?

Jim's Story

For many years, Jim had encountered this danger firsthand.

Jim had 20/20 vision. His eyesight had always been 20/20. As a child in the pediatrician's office, his eyesight had been 20/20. Year after year during school screenings his eyesight had been 20/20. Even in elementary school, when he had complained to his mother that he was having trouble seeing to read, a trip to the eye doctor had revealed that Jim's eyesight was 20/20.

When the eye doctor told him that there was "nothing the matter with his eyes" Jim began to wonder if his trouble seeing was in his mind. Rather than be ridiculed by another doctor, Jim quit complaining. For this reason, he struggled through over half a decade of school without anyone suspecting the truth about his vision: he could not read more than 10 minutes before the print began to blur and run together.

Because of his vision problem, Jim could not stick with his reading. He would begin reading well enough, but within a few minutes his mind would start wandering and he would develop an urge to get away from the book. If he continued to read, his eyes would start to bother him and eventually he would begin to see the print blur and double. Rather than endure the frustration, Jim learned to avoid reading whenever possible.

Being intelligent, Jim would listen in class carefully and do well when tested on any material which the teacher covered verbally. Also, because math does not require the same sustained visual effort demanded by reading, Jim did well in math, except on story problems. Despite his success in school, however, Jim's self-confidence was secretly low because he knew he couldn't read like his friends.

In high school Jim was finally referred to our

office by one of the ever increasing number of optometrists who understand that there are vision problems which affect reading but have nothing to do with 20/20 eyesight.

The referring doctor had found that Jim's eyes were healthy and that he did not require glasses to see 20/20. We performed an additional set of tests which are not part of the routine eye examination. These tests revealed that Jim had a vision problem which was unrelated to Snellen's 1862 eye chart. For this reason the problem—which explained Jim's inability to read without blurred and double vision—had been previously overlooked.

Four months later, after treatment for his condition, Jim was able to read for over an hour at a time without blurred or double vision or loss of comprehension. Now that his vision no longer served as a road block, he began to read for pleasure. The more he read, the better he became until college posed no problem for him. At the end of six years he had received his Masters of Business Administration degree!

The Most Dangerous Assumption

Unlike many other children with similar vision problems, Jim's story had a happy ending. For Jim, however, 20/20 had been a real danger—to his reading, his education, and his self-esteem.

The danger did not lie in his ability to read tiny

letters at twenty feet. The danger was to be found in his parent's—and the first doctor's—assumption that 20/20 eyesight is enough for good school performance. Indeed, this is the most dangerous assumption that you, as a parent, can make about your child's vision.

Traditions die hard. But no matter how many "authorities" have told you that "20/20 is perfect vision," Snellen's 1862 eye chart is no longer the beginning and end of vision testing.

This advance is especially important for children because they seldom tell others about what they are seeing, or even realize that blurred and double vision are abnormal. For this reason it is CRUCIAL that you understand the following:

20/20 means only that your child can see tiny letters across the room FOR AS LONG AS IT TAKES TO READ THE EYE CHART.

20/20 does not mean that your child can see the chalkboard at the end of the day when he is tired. It does not mean that your child can see to read without blurred or double vision. It does not mean that he can use his eyes to guide a pencil when writing. It does not mean that he can control his eyes well enough to keep his place when reading. It does not mean that he can understand or remember the distorted information coming in through his eyes. In short, 20/20 eyesight is absolutely NO guarantee that your child has the visual abilities to succeed in school!

Visual Abilities Defined

But what do we mean by "visual abilities"?

An ability may be defined as "the power or means to do something." *Visual abilities* are the skills which give us the power or means to locate, identify and remember what we see. The best known visual ability is that of seeing tiny letters in the distance; that is, "20/20 Acuity."

In addition to 20/20 *acuity*, there are a number of other visual abilities which are necessary for your child to perform at potential in school. These abilities include keeping things clear at different distances (including reading distance), keeping things from going double, judging depth, locating words when reading, guiding a pencil, recognizing what is seen, and remembering what is seen.

Without these abilities school can become a struggle for your child and a source of frustration and unhappiness for both your child and yourself. To give you the understanding to avoid this frustration and unhappiness, the remaining chapters in this section of the book will describe the various visual abilities which your child needs to succeed in school. The chapters will also provide you with information to help detect if your child is missing any of these abilities.

CHAPTER 6

The Child Who "Just Wanted Glasses"

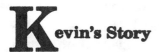evin's Story

When Kevin entered fourth grade, the pages contained more words and the print grew smaller and smaller. Gradually he began struggling to keep things clear. Sometimes Kevin could see the words on the chalkboard distinctly; other times the same words would blur in and out of focus. When Kevin read, he would encounter the same frustration: the print would alternate between being clear one minute and blurred the next.

We have only so much effort available. As Kevin put more and more of that effort into seeing clearly, he had less and less effort left over with which to understand what he was seeing. As a result, when report cards came out, Kevin's grades dropped sharply, especially in subjects such as social studies and science which depended on reading.

When Kevin's mother asked him if anything was wrong, he finally explained that he was having trouble seeing. Being a concerned parent, she immediately asked a friend for the name of an eye doctor and arranged an appointment.

During the examination, Kevin was nervous at first and could not see to read the smaller letters on the doctor's eye chart. The letters blurred in and out, just like they did in the afternoons at school. This time, however, Kevin was not concerned about the blurred letters and did not struggle to clear them. He assummed that the doctor would give him glasses that would "fix" his eyes.

As Kevin's mother watched the examination, it appeared to her that the doctor looked puzzled. Finally, he demanded that Kevin try harder to read the chart and waited somewhat impatiently as Kevin slowly called out each letter, still making occassional errors.

When the doctor had finished his measurements, he turned to Kevin's mother and told her that there was "nothing wrong with Kevin's eyes." He went on to explain that Kevin's eyes were healthy and that he did not need glasses.

When Kevin's mother asked why her son had so

much trouble reading the chart, the doctor told her, "He probably just wants glasses." Kevin listened in disbelief to the doctor's words.

Fortunately for Kevin, his mother was in the habit of telling the truth herself, so it did not seem likely to her that her son was fibbing to "get glasses." Therefore, instead of listening to the doctor, she decided to get a second opinion.

This time, before deciding on a doctor, Kevin's mother spoke to a number of parents about Kevin's previous examination and the discrepancy between her child's symptoms and the doctor's findings. Finally she found a parent whose child had complained of similar problems despite "20/20 eyesight." This parent directed Kevin and his mother to us.

When we examined Kevin, we initially found the same findings that the first doctor had found: healthy eyes and no glasses that would improve Kevin's vision. Additional testing, however, which is usually not part of the general eye examination, revealed that Kevin had a difficulty of a different kind.

The Reason

As covered in Chapter 4, when a child who does not need glasses looks at a distant object, light enters the eye through the *pupil*, passes through the *lens* of the eye and is focused on the *retina* of the eye (Figure 1).

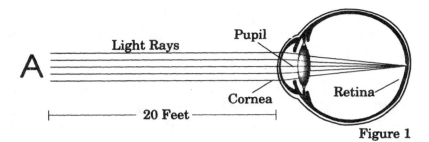

Figure 1

If the same child next looks at a book which is closer than the distant object, the light entering the eye will now be focused behind the retina (Figure 2).

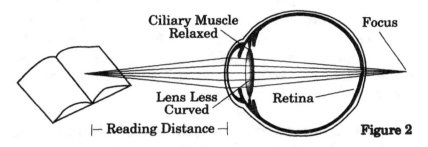

Figure 2

To compensate for the defocused light, the child must tighten his *ciliary muscle* to make the lens more curved and refocus the light on the retina (Figure 3).

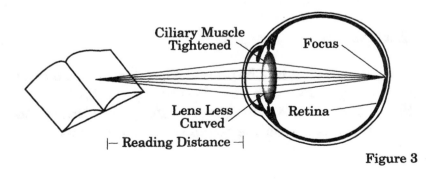

Figure 3

In summary then, just as a camera must be "refocused" to take clear pictures at different distances, so must a child accurately "adjust" his eyes to see clearly at different distances. We call this ability to change the shape of the lens of the eye to focus things at different distances *accommodation*. The word *accommodation* comes from the Latin word which means "to adapt." When we *accommodate*, we adapt our vision to see at some desired distance. To see clearly far away, we relax accommodation. To see clearly at reading distance or closer, we increase accommodation.

In Kevin's case, he was having difficulty accurately controlling accommodation. For this reason, things were clear one minute and blurred the next. Although for Kevin there were no glasses that would correct his condition, there was a program of therapy which allowed Kevin to regain this ability to keep things clear. After completing the program, Kevin no longer suffered from blurred vision. More importantly, his grades improved and he rediscovered the joy of reading—much to his mother's relief.

The Three Abilities

Unfortunately for children like Kevin, a routine eye examination generally does not include a thorough evaluation of accommodation. Such an evaluation needs to consider three separate abilities:

The first ability to be considered is the the *power* of accommodation. The closer to his eyes that a child can clearly see, the more powerful is his accommodation.

A second ability is *flexibility* of accommodation. The quicker that a child can see clearly when shifting attention from one distance to another, the more *flexible* is his accommodation.

A third and possibly most important ability is *maintenance* of accommodation. The longer that a child can look at the same distance and continue to see clearly without experiencing any momentary blurring of vision, the better is his ability to *maintain* accommodation.

The power of accommodation is generally lost between the ages of 45 and 50 as a normal part of growing older. Because of this loss of focusing ability with age, all eye-care practitioners measure the *power* of accommodation in patients in the "over-forty" range.

Unlike the power of accommodation, however, the flexibility and maintenance of accommodation do not necessarily wait to break down until a person reaches his forties. As a result, deficits in flexiblity and maintenance are frequently overlooked during routine eye examinations of children.

The three accommodative abilities are important for all of us at any age, but they are critical for your child's performance at school.

To easily shift focus between chalkboard and desk,

one must have good flexibility of accommodation. If such flexibilty is lacking, your child will experience momentary blurred vision when shifting from one distance to another. The time wasted waiting for the things to clear results in boardwork assignments taking too long to complete. The harder the child works, the longer it takes for things to clear, and the more schoolwork is left to be completed at home.

As accommodation is fatigued, the ability to maintain clear vision may be reduced. At this point your child may be bothered by the print blurring in and out as he reads or looks at the chalkboard. The blurring may contribute to "careless errors" caused by the struggle to interpret half-clear print.

Worse than the blurring, however, is the fatigue which results from the effort used to overcome the problem and maintain clarity. When reading, the child with a maintenance problem begins much better than he finishes. He sits down to read and very soon begins to feel as if he would "like to be somewhere else." At this point his attention becomes difficult to maintain and he has to work harder and harder to "make sense" out of what he is reading. He, therefore, has to reread sentences. It is almost as if he is "smart" for a page or two and then becomes a little "stupider" with each page he reads; even BEFORE the print blurs, this difficulty with reading comprehension has already begun.

The continual effort to clear things is likely to cause sore eyes and headaches or, more commonly, avoid ance of the task; it is easier to talk to a friend than to struggle against blurred vision. It is easier to quickly glance at schoolwork than to carefully view each detail. As a result your child may even be incorrectly labeled as having a problem with "behavior" or "attention."

Because the problem increases as fatigue sets in, the child who failed to complete work in school experiences even more difficulty at the end of an already long day when requested to complete the work at home. Such children would prefer to do almost anything rather than labor over more deskwork. As a result, homework may drag on for hours and lead you and your child to feel more like adversaries than friends.

The Eight Signs of an Accommodation Problem

As a parent, what are clues which should lead you to suspect that your child may have difficulty with the ability to keep things clear? The following is a list of some behaviors which could be related to such a difficulty.

1. Reading comprehension is good when your child first begins reading but then rapidly reduces the longer reading is continued. Your child begins reading well, but all too rapidly begins to squirm and want to get away.

2. Your child avoids reading. Pages are counted before reading commences and only shorter works are attempted.

3. Your child complains of discomfort about the eyes or headaches when reading. Younger children, rather than complaining, may rub their eyes or merely avoid reading.

4. Your child blinks excessively when reading or looking at street signs or the chalkboard as if trying to "clear things up."

5. Your child complains that things are blurry even though a vision screening or eye examination has demonstrated 20/20 acuity.

6. Your child holds books too close to his eyes or moves the book or his head closer and further away as if to clear things.

7. Your child makes seemingly careless errors when reading or copying from the chalkboard. Long words like *rhinoceros* are recognized while little words such as *of*, *as*, and *is*, or small beginnings and endings of words are misread or confused.

8. Your child's reading comprehension is not as good as his intelligence would predict. Math, with the exception of "story problems," is better than subjects such as English, social studies, or science, which require reading. The more reading there is to do, the worse the problem becomes.

The Questions to Ask your Child

Any ONE of the above listed behaviors could signal that your child is having difficulty with accommodation. Another techinique which is useful in helping to determine if a problem exists is to ASK your child the following questions:

1. When you're reading, do the words ever "blur" or look fuzzy for a second? Do the words ever get "hard to see?"

2. When you are reading and you first look up at the chalkboard, are the words ever blurry or fuzzy for a second or two?

For a younger child who may not understand what the word "blurred" means, or the child who habitually gets away from reading before the onset of the blur, or a child who is afraid of getting glasses, these two questions may not turn up any evidence of a problem with accommodation—even when such a problem exists.

If, however, your child is old enough to understand your questions and does not completely avoid reading, a "yes" response to either of the two questions is good evidence that a problem exists—no matter what a school screening or a routine eye examination discloses.

In working with thousands of children over the

past decade who have "perfect eyes," it has been my experience that children seldom lie about blurred vision solely to get glasses. While it is true that many children will exaggerate the severity of the blur—possibly to both themselves and the examiner—they do so in the hopes that their problems will not be missed. The exagerations are a "cry for help." When the ability to keep things clear is restored, these children not only see more clearly, they are happier and perform better in both school and sports.

Based on this experience, I would make a firm recommendation to every parent: listen to your child and do not stop listening no matter what any professional tells you. Even though increasing numbers of doctors across the nation are beginnng to recognize that 20/20 eyesight is not "perfect vision," there are still many who do not check for other visual abilities than 20/20. As a parent, then, your best strategy is to continue to ask, look, and listen until your child's problems are resolved. More will be said on this subject in this book's third section, *Finding Help*.

Glasses

Sometimes it will be found during a routine eye examination that a child who appears to have difficulty with accommodation may need glasses. These glasses may or may not solve the problem. For this reason, even if glasses are prescribed, it will still be necessary for you, as a parent, to be certain that your child does not continue to exhibit any of the Eight Signs of an

Accommodation Problem when wearing the new glasses. If these signs continue, then additional testing is definitely indicated.

Summary

Even the child with 20/20 eyesight during a vision screening or general eye examination may nonetheless be struggling to overcome blurred vision in school. In all cases, this struggle will cause your child to perform below potential. In some cases, the struggle may be too great and defeat both your child and you. Being aware of the Eight Signs of an Accommodation Problem and seeking help until these problems are solved is your best defense against your child's frustration and failure.

Drill

If you already wear bifocals because of your age, then you are personally aware of what effect an accommodation problem can have on your reading. If, however, you can still see clearly at reading distance, the following drill will help you to understand accommodation.

Look at the face of your watch. Move the watch as close to your eyes as you possibly can without the watch face blurring. Leave the watch in this position for the rest of this drill. Now look far away at something in the distance until it clears up. Again, look at the watch face AS CLOSE TO YOUR EYES AS YOU CAN BARELY CLEAR IT. Again, look far away and clear things in the distance. Continue working near-far-near-far until your eyes fatigue.

During this drill, each time you look at the watch face you are increasing accommodation; each time you look far away you are relaxing accommodation. Providing that you hold the watch as close as you are barely able to clear it, the way you will begin to feel as your eyes fatigue is the way a child with a decreased accommodation ability feels whenever he reads. It is small wonder that many such children avoid reading whenever possible.

CHAPTER 7

When The Words Run Together

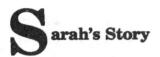arah's Story

In fourth grade when the print had grown smaller and reading was required in every subject, Sarah began to dislike reading. Being a good student, she continued to work and study, but when she did read, her eyes would hurt and she would get headaches. After she had read several pages, her mind would wander and she would have to reread sentences several times to understand them. From that time on, Sarah no longer read for fun.

From time to time Sarah's mother would take her to an eye doctor in the hope that a reason for Sarah's avoidance of reading would be found. At the time of the first exam, a doctor had concluded that Sarah had no vision problem which would affect reading. Several years later, a second doctor had prescribed reading glasses. Sarah had felt that the glasses definitely helped reduce the number of headaches, but she still could not comfortably read for more than fifteen or twenty minutes. Finally, when Sarah was fifteen years old, a third doctor had listened to Sarah's symptoms, found that glasses would not relieve her problem, and referred her to us.

In talking to Sarah before beginning her testing, she told me that the print would blur when she read—with or without her glasses. She went on to say that she would get headaches which began around her eyes whenever she read. In response to a question I asked, she shared one more bit of information which no matter how often I hear, I am always amazed: when Sarah read, the words would pull apart and run together.

Now, what amazes me, is not that children see double. There is an explanation for double vision which we will cover in detail in this chapter. Nor is double vision uncommon. If the truth be known, there are probably two children in every classroom who, when they read, see double.

What amazes me is that in asking over three dozen children who lacked the ability to keep the print single, "Have you ever told anyone that the words pull apart?" only two of the thirty-six children surveyed had mentioned the problem to anyone! Indeed when I asked Sarah—age fifteen— if she had ever told anyone about her double vision, she turned to her mother and asked, "Mom, don't you see the words run together?"

Imagine how Sarah felt! Imagine how her mother felt!

Up to that point, it had never occurred to Sarah that double vision was abnormal. She had been seeing double for over five years and she felt the whole world saw that way! Five years of seeing the words "dance," five years of avoiding reading, five years of frustration, five years of wasted effort, and Sarah, like thousands of other children bearing every label under the educational sun, moon, and stars, had not shared her real problem with a soul.

If she had not finally stumbled across a family optometrist who understood that seeing to read requires more than 20/20 eyesight, Sarah, like countless adults in every community, might have gone through life feeling inadequate—if not stupid—because reading came so hard. Once Sarah's problem was identified, it took but several months to teach her the ability to keep the print single. After that, not only did her headaches and double vision disappear, she was able to enjoy reading for the first time in half a decade.

That children like Sarah should have to silently suffer is a tragedy—both for the children themselves and for the parents who suffer with them! It is time that every parent knew how to prevent stories like Sarah's from happening.

The Cause of Double Vision

There are few parts of the body which must work together with more precision than the eyes. Imagine how difficult it would be, even for five minutes, to perfectly coordinate your arms so that when one moved any distance up, down, left or right, the other arm moved EXACTLY the same distance in EXACTLY the same direction. Imagine next, that every time one arm trailed even a sixteenth of an inch behind the other that you would see double. Well, this is the precision with which the two eyes must function together to avoid double vision—not just for five minutes at a time, but all day long.

We call this ability to maintain both eyes pointed at precisely the same object (or the same word or letter in the case of reading) *eye teaming*. Eye teaming is a crucial ability for your child to have in order to perform without frustration in school. When both eyes are accurately aimed at the object being viewed the information coming from the two eyes will be combined in the mind in a single image (Figure 1).

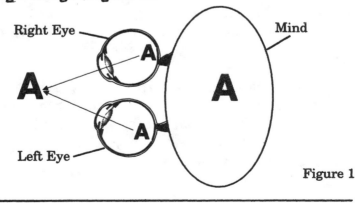

Right Eye

Left Eye

Mind

Figure 1

If, however, one eye is aimed at the object being viewed and the other eye is pointed even a fraction of an inch to the side, the information from the two eyes will not be correctly combined in the mind and double vision will occur (Figure 2).

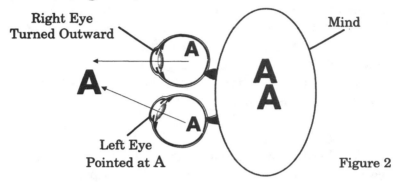

Figure 2

The further one eye is aimed to one side, the further apart the double images will be perceived. The child with an obviously crossed eye, for instance, may—if the mind has not learned to ignore all information coming in through the turned eye—see "two books" when reading. Because crossed eyes are generally obvious to the examiner, such problems are seldom over-looked during a routine eye exam.

For the child, however, whose eyes are aligned but slip almost imperceptable amounts when that child reads,· the words may not even pull entirely apart. Rather, the letters may merely run together. Figure 3 is a represenation of the print doubling due to one eye

The dog ran home

Figure 3

turning so slightly that someone watching the child would be unable to see anything abnormal about that child's eyes.

The smaller the print being viewed, the more noticeable double vision becomes. When reading the headlines in a newspaper, for instance, if one eye were to slip very slightly, the print would probably not appear to double. If, however, a child is looking at print in a book, the tiniest misalignment of the two eyes can result in double vision.

Learning to read is difficult enough when the words always look the same way. When words look one way one moment and then double up in an ever-changing and unpredictable fashion the next, learning to read can become a nightmare.

For most children who experience double vision when reading, however, their problem revolves less around the confusion caused by the double vision than around the effort expended to avoid the double vision. As do children who lack *accommodation* ability, children who lack eye teaming ability, rapidly fatigue and lose comprehension as they continue reading. The harder they try, the more things double and the more difficult reading becomes.

How to Detect Double Vision

As a parent, what are the signs which might suggest that your child has difficulty with eye teaming ability? For the most part any of the signs which appear in Chapter 6 regarding accommodation could also signal the presense of double vision which some children merely interpret as a different form of "blurred" vision. Some additional signs of deficient eye teaming abilities include the following:

Seven Signs of Deficient Eye Teaming Ability

1. Your child covers or closes one eye when reading.

2. Your child tends to rest his head on the palm of one hand when reading. The hand "just happens" to cover one eye.

3. Your child holds the book to one side or turns his head to one side when reading so that both eyes cannot see the print at the same time.

4. Your child adds or removes parts from words when reading.

5. When copying materials from the chalkboard, your child repeats letters within words.

6. When performing math problems, your child fails to align the columns of numbers correctly because the numbers are seen to run together.

7. Your child demonstrates any of the signs given on pages 68-69 of Chapter 6 of this book.

Sometimes, but not always, questioning your child can provide you with information concerning the presence of double vision. The way the questions are asked, however, can limit their usefulness. If, for example, you ask your child, "Do you see double when you read?" most children will not understand what you are talking about and will answer, "No." A better method is to ask if the words ever "pull apart or run together?"

Possibly the best method to explain to a child what you mean about double vision is to do a demonstration with your hands. First, with your fingers spread apart, place your palms together so that your fingers are superimposed (Figure 4). Next, with the back of one of your hands facing your child, ask him if when he reads the words ever run together like "this?" As you say the word "this" slide your hands slightly until your spread fingers are alongside one another rather than superimposed (Figure 5).

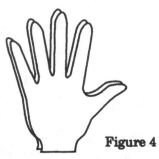
Figure 4

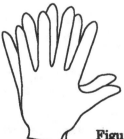
Figure 5

Even though most children will at first deny seeing double, when they are shown this demonstration, they are likely to immediately nod their heads with recognition of what you are asking.

Summary

Outside of visual acuity itself, accommodation and eye teaming are the two most important visual abilities required for your child to succeed to potential in school. If accommodation is deficient, your child will have to struggle to keep things clear. If eye teaming ability is deficient, your child will have to struggle to avoid double vision. These struggles can cause headaches, uncomfortable eyes, loss of comprehension when reading and even difficulty learning how to read. While a routine eye examination may reveal if your child's eyes are crossed or if glasses are needed to see the chalkboard, such an exam will normally not detect any of the more subtle reasons for blurred or double vision. For this reason you should be familiar with the signs of these "hidden" vision problems so that they do not become major obstacles to your child's education.

What can be done for double vision and where to turn for help for this problem will be covered in the third section of this book.

CHAPTER 8

The Lost Child

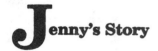

Jenny's Story

"Look at the doctor, Jenny, when he's talking to you!" When Jenny's mother voiced these words, she was not giving a command so much as expressing a wish. She wished that her daughter had the skills to be happy in life. She knew how important the ability to comfortably talk to others would be in every area of her daughter's life. She was, therefore, concerned when her daughter failed to maintain the eye contact which is so necessary for good communication.

Jenny's mother, however, had not brought Jenny in because of difficulty with eye contact. Instead, the reason for the visit were the tears of frustration which Jenny's work in school brought on. Jenny's mother had found us through a long-time friend of hers whose child had suffered with similar frustration.

In school, Jenny encountered persistent problems with learning how to read. She would frequently lose her place, omit or insert small words, skip or accidentally reread sentences, or use her finger to keep her place.

Watching Jenny read was kind of like watching a chicken pecking the keys of a typewriter: rather than turn just her eyes, Jenny would bob her entire head when moving from word to word. It almost looked as if she were keeping her place by pointing her nose—rather than her eyes—at the words. As a result, she read haltingly, "one - word - at - a - time," with a pause in between each word.

In addition, Jenny hated doing boardwork. Each time she looked from her paper back up to the board, she had to painstakingly search to refind her place. For this reason, she rapidly became frustrated and fidgety. After struggling with this activity for a short while, she found it easier to stare out the window—LOST.

Indeed, Jenny was lost. She was lost when she read, lost when she did boardwork, lost in school and lost when you spoke to her. The reason? She did not have the visual ability needed to know where she was pointing her eyes. She would think her eyes were pointed one place when they were actually pointed somewhere else. The end result of this missing visual ability was confusion—for Jenny, her teachers, and her mother.

Eye Movment Ability Defined

In Chapter 7, we discussed an ability where the two eyes have to work together to point in the same spot to avoid double vision. We called that ability *eye teaming*.

In Jenny's case, the problem was not getting her two eyes to work together, the problem was to teach her accurately to track with her eyes when looking from one point to another. We call this visual ability *eye movements*. Children need good eye movement whether they are keeping their eyes on the ball in sports or looking from word to word when reading. Unless eye movements are accurate, mistakes will be made.

This observation is based on a simple fact: if you are not looking directly at something, you cannot really see it.

The reason for this fact concerns the way the eye is built. As covered in Chapter 3, the "movie screen" on the back of the inside of the eye is called the *retina*.

The retina is divided into two regions. There is a tiny central region called the *fovea* which sends millions of messages to the brain and which is responsible for our clear, central vision. There is also a peripheral area of the retina which sends far fewer messages to the brain and which is responsible for our less clear peripheral vision (Figure 1).

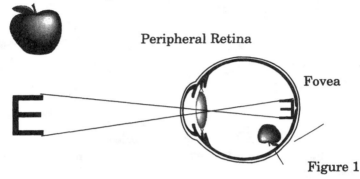

Figure 1

Objects which are located above, below, or to the side of where the eye is pointed (such as the apple in Figure 1) are imaged on the peripheral retina and cannot be seen clearly. Objects which are directly in front of where the eye is pointing (such as the "E" in Figure 1) are focused on the *fovea*. Such objects (or print) can be seen clearly.

To observe for yourself how your central vision is better than your peripheral vision, try this experiment: Look at this asterisk * and see how many words to the side of the asterisk you can clearly see without moving your eye.

The reason the asterisk is clear and the words to the side are blurry is because your foveas are directed at the asterisk and your peripheral retina is "seeing" the words.

As you can see from this experiment, we have only a tiny area of clear central vision. Our peripheral vision is indistinct. For this reason, it is of supreme importance for your child to have good *eye movements* in order to point his eyes in a manner which allows the images of words being viewed to be accurately aligned on his foveas. If eye movements are slow, reading and schoolwork will be slow. If eye movements are inaccurate, vision will be inaccurate and your child will make seemingly "careless" errors.

In Jenny's case, she had difficulty with eye movements. As a result she could not maintain her place when reading. We worked with Jenny over several months to teach her this ability. When we finished, her reading was much smoother and she had far less trouble completing assigments on time. From her mother's standpoint, however, the most important improvement was that now Jenny could maintain eye contact when carrying on a conversation.

The Five Signs of Deficient Eye Movement Abilities

As a parent what are the signs which might lead you to suspect that your child is having difficulty with eye movement ability? The following list contains five signs any ONE of which could suggest a problem with eye movements:

1. Your child moves his head rather than his eyes when reading.

2. Your child too frequently loses his place or skips lines when reading.

3. Your child makes seemingly careless errors when reading. Beginnings or endings of words are altered or missed. "Small" words are skipped.

4. Past the age of seven, your child needs a finger to keep his place when reading.

5. Your child is labelled as having a problem with "attention."

Screening for Eye Movement Problems

While there are not really any questions which you can ask your child to reveal a problem with eye movements, there is a simple screening which you can perform: First have your child call out the numbers in Screening Test One (at the end of this chapter) in a left to right fashion as quickly as he can. Thus, he should call out "seven, four, eight, six, two, nine, six, four, eight, one," etc., as quickly as possible. Let him practice Test One several times until he understands the test and can get through it.

Next, have your child do Screening Test Two one time. This time, as you can see, the numbers are not connected. You will, therefore, have to explain to your child how you want him to read "straight across" each line without skipping to the next line. Also, show your child with your finger what you mean.

Finally, use a stop watch or a watch with a second hand to time your child as he reads through the numbers as quickly as he can. Record in seconds how long it takes to complete all forty numbers.

If you have any concerns that your child did not perform at potential, repeat the screening on a different day.

Accuracy

This test should not be performed with children under age six because it will only frustrate them.

A six-year-old is expected to skip one or two lines when reading the numbers. A seven-year-old is expected to skip one line. Age eight and older children should not add or skip more than one or two numbers. If your child is age 6 or older and cannot perform the test or if he skips more numbers than expected for his age then there is an indication of possible difficulties with eye movement abilities.

Expected Times

As children become older, they typically take less time to finish reading the 40 numbers in this test. The following table gives average times for a given age group of children. If your child takes longer than the times given in Table # 1 then he is performing below average for his age. For instance, an average seven-year-old should take about 45 seconds to complete the test. If your seven-year-old takes 50 or 60 seconds to complete the test, then we can suspect that he is having a tougher than average time for his age with eye movements.

Table # 1

Age	Time in Seconds
6	50
7	45
8 through 10	30
11 and older	20

Obviously, this test is only a crude screening test. Failure on this screening in no way "proves" that your child is having trouble with eye movements any more than passing this screening proves that your child has perfect eye movement abilities. The screening merely gives you an impression of how your child compares to others his age in the area of eye movements.

Whether or not your child passes this screening, if you are seeing any of the "Five Signs of Deficient Eye Movement Abilities," then a full evaluation by a doctor who works with improving eye movement ability is definitely indicated.

Summary

If your child has difficulty with finding his place

when reading or doing boardwork, there is a good chance that his eye movement abilities are deficient. Fortunately—as we will see in a later chapter—eye movement abilities are trainable so that your child will not have to continue to experience this frustration.

Eye-Movement Screening Test One

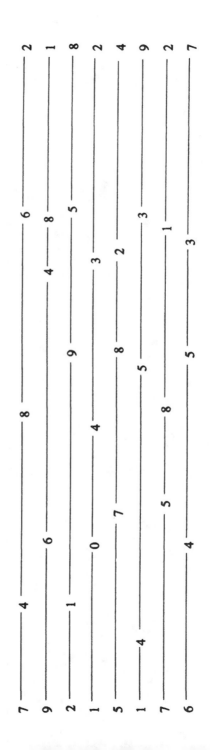

Eye-Movement Screening Test Two

```
5    4   7     8     2   3   4

1        4      5         3       9

7    4       5   8        6       2

6                9     4       7   7

8    3       5         1

5    3       9     4       5       2

2    1       7         4   7       8

1    0       3         3   5       9
```

CHAPTER 9

The Child Who
Saw Backwards

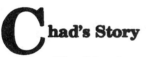had's Story

Chad had completed kindergarten for the second time and was now seven and scheduled to begin first grade. He was a good-natured little boy who tried hard and he had a mother who tried just as hard to help him. Despite both their best efforts, however, Chad still had difficulty recognizing the alphabet. No matter how often he and his mother practiced, he still could not tell a "b" from a "d". When he did write, he frequently wrote the letters as if he were seeing them backwards.

Because of his difficulty in school, Chad's mother had brought him to eye doctors both when Chad was age five and six. Each examination had revealed that Chad had healthy eyes and did not need glasses to see the chalkboard.

With the beginning of first grade approaching, Chad would already be one of the tallest children in his class. His mother was rightly concerned about Chad's lack of progress; she certainly did not want to see him have to repeat first grade as well. For this reason when a school counselor—who fortunately knew about vision's role in learning—suggested Chad see us, Chad's mother wasted no time in making an appointment.

We saw Chad in August just before school started. We found, as had the other doctors, that Chad would not benefit from glasses. Additional testing, however, showed that Chad lacked the ability to "understand" the information entering his eyes. He could not compare things and see how they were different. We call this ability to understand what is seen *visual perception.*

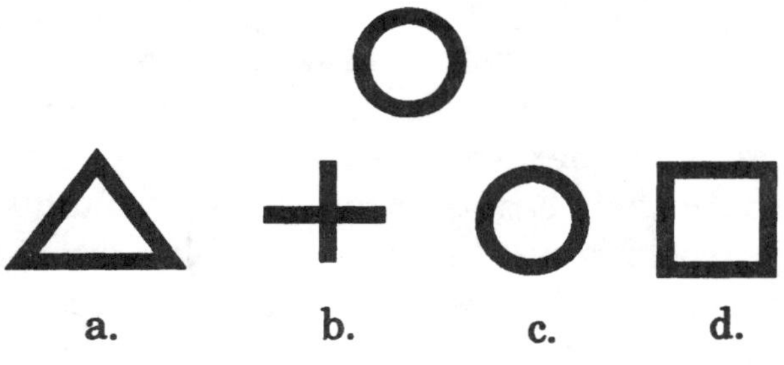

a.   b.   c.   d.

Figure 1

Figures 1 through 3 are examples of visual perception. In a test made up of figures which are similar to these, a child is asked to find which one of the bottom four forms matches the top form. In Figure 1, for instance, "Form C" matches the "circle" above. The child who lacks the ability to tell the difference between a "circle," "square," "triangle," and "cross" is quite obviously not ready to learn his letters. He might not even be able to tell the difference between the letter "t" which resembles a cross and the letter "O" which resembles a circle.

In Figure 2, the upper form is composed of a vertical line intersected by two horizontal lines; one horizontal line intersects the "top" of the vertical line; the other horizontal line intersects the "center" of the vertical line. Choice "B" below matches the upper form. In choice A the "top" line has been shifted to the "bottom." In choice "C" there are "three" horizontal lines instead of "two." In choice "D" one of the horizontal lines has been shifted from the "center" to the "bottom" of the vertical line.

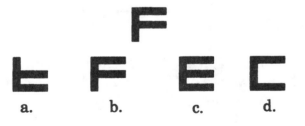

a.   b.   c.   d.

Figure 2

To "see" to perform this task, the child would, therefore, need at least some understanding of such concepts as "top, bottom, and center" as well as to be able to tell the difference between "three and two." If he did not understand these concepts, he might write his "F's" upside down or confuse his "F's" with his "E's".

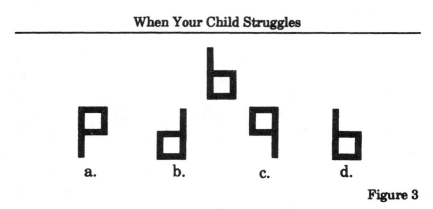

a.   b.   c.   d.

Figure 3

In Figure 3 to match the form on top with "Choice D" on the bottom, the child would have to know how to compare the directions which the forms are pointing. In this figure, the "squares" vary as to how they are connected to the vertical lines. In "C" the square is on the "top" and "left-hand" side of the vertical line. In "D" the square is on the "bottom" and "right-hand" side. To answer questions such as this one correctly on a consistent basis, a child would have to understand the difference between "top and bottom," as well as the difference between "left and right."

Remember, in the English language when we say, "I see," we mean "I understand." The child who has difficulty with the ability of visual perception does not really understand so he cannot really "see." This lack of understanding is the reason why children who cannot match forms such as those in Figure 3 frequently appear to "see backwards" and cannot tell the difference between "b's" and "d's" or "was" and "saw". They are not really "seeing backward;" they are merely confused.

This confusion was the reason why Chad was

having difficulty conquering the alphabet. Fortunately for Chad, the ability of visual preception, like other visual abilities, is in some cases trainable. By the time fall had passed and Christmas was approaching, Chad had worked hard and had a special "gift" for his mother: not only could he read the alphabet, he was beginning to recognize words as well.

With the help of a reading tutor, who could now go back and fill in what was missed before Chad "learned to see," Chad went on to learn to read, pass first grade, and grow in confidence and ability. The tragedy of years of needless struggle and frustration was averted by early visual intervention.

Signs of a Visual Perception Problem

As a parent what should lead you to suspect that your child has difficulty with the ability of visual perception? Any of the following six signs, if present, might signal the presence of such a problem:

1. Your child is not learning how to read on schedule. He is having difficulty learning to recognize words.

2. Your child is having difficulty in kindergarten.

3. Your child is still having problems recognizing letters or numbers past the end of kindergarten.

4. Your child is still writing "b's" and "d's" backwards past the end of first grade (It is normal for kindergarten students to "reverse" letters. By the end of first grade, however, only about two out of ten children are still reversing.)

5. Your child frequently confuses similar beginnings or endings of words.

6. Your child recognizes the sounds of individual letters but cannot break words down into syllables so as to "sound them out."

Summary

Visual perception is the ability to understand and recognize likes and differences in what is seen. For your child to successfully learn how to read, this visual ability must be present. If your child demonstrates any of the above "signs," he could be suffering from deficient ability with visual perception. Once the seriousness of the problem is determined by an evaluation which tests for more than just 20/20 eyesight, then decisions can be made on how best to help your child.

CHAPTER 10

If Only He Could Get His Thoughts on Paper

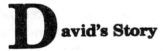avid's Story

David was definitely a bright child. Talking to him throughout his examination left no doubt in my mind. He answered questions easily, accurately, and without hesitation. He could immediately see how different parts of his examination were related to one another. Most importantly, when I explained to David how his vision was affecting him, he completely understood—for the first time in his life—why he was so miserable in school. As his parent's listened, they also understood the reason for the fights with David at home which were gradually eroding their relationship with their son.

David's problem in sixth grade was that his written work was either sloppy or incomplete. Testing, performed by the school, had demonstrated that David was quite intelligent—a fact that was well supported by his excellent participation in classroom discussions and his reading ability, which was several years ahead of his classmates.

Despite this "superior intelligence," however, David continued to turn in assignments in which the writing was crooked, poorly spaced, off the lines, full of "careless" errors and generally unacceptable. Try as he would, he could not get his thoughts down on paper.

Nor was composition the only subject affected. David's math was often so sloppy that he misaligned columns, added the wrong numbers, and failed to get credit for his work even though he understood the concepts. During spelling tests he would leave out letters in words that he had easily spelled for his mother the night before. It made no sense.

Occasionally, the teacher would convince David to "take his time." During such instances his handwriting was much neater, proving to both David's teachers and his parents that he could do it if he would "just apply himself." For this reason, both in school and at home, all David heard was,"You're much too bright to be turning in work which looks like this!"

Gradually David started not turning in his assignments at all. His grades fell. When neither bribes nor threats, anger nor sympathy reversed this trend, his parents finally began to suspect that something else was wrong; their son's conduct was more and more a puzzle to them, and it appeared that a piece of the puzzle was missing.

When we examined David, we found the missing piece of the puzzle. Although he had 20/20 eyesight he, nonetheless, had difficulty with the ability of getting his eyes to guide his hands. We call this visual ability, *eye-hand coordination.*

Children who lack ability in the area of eye-hand coordination have difficulty with controlling a pencil. So much "thinking" goes into moving the pencil that little remains for neatness, accuracy, or just getting the thoughts down on the page. It is almost as if there is a "short circuit" between the eyes and hands. No matter how quickly the mind moves, the hands cannot keep pace.

Because of these characteristics, such a child is left with two choices; he can either write very slowly and carefully and, as a result, not finish assignments, or he can finish on time at the expense of legibility. In the first case, he is penalized with excessive homework, in the second case, he is labeled as "careless" or "sloppy." Either way, he loses.

If the child with poor eye-hand coordination is a "slow" thinker, teachers may attribute the "sloppy" hand-writing to retarded development in all areas and not call undue attention to the handwriting problem. If, however, the child has the misfortune of being verbally bright and of showing "high intelligence," then all concerned are likely to confuse the sloppy penmanship with "lack of effort," a "behavior problem," or even a problem with "attention."

If a child with poor eye-hand coordination is lucky, his teacher will consider neatness only in the subject of "handwriting," and not count off in other subjects because of crooked writing. If, however, a teacher considers neatness in every subject, then the child with the eye-hand coordination problem will be penalized in every subject. No matter what he really knows in English, social studies, science, and spelling, his report card will reflect merely his handwriting ability, not his understanding of the material.

If your child is placed in this situation, school can become a real nightmare. Imagine being in a footrace in which you are submerged up to your chest in water and your competitors are allowed to run on dry land. Imagine the frustration of running this race all day in school and then coming home to run the race again when you do homework. It is small wonder that some children rebel.

Such was the case with David. Although he was highly intelligent, our testing showed that this 12-year-old boy had the eye-hand coordination ability of an eight-year old. As soon as he and his parents and his teachers understood that "his hands were not as quick as his mind," David's frustration level dropped tremendously. Rather than center all their attention on his handwriting, all concerned (including David himself) began to appreciate David for his strengths.

Now this is not to say that we suggested to David that he do less than his best or that he had a problem "he would have to learn to live with." Instead, we worked with David to improve his eye-hand coordination ability. Gradually, as this visual ability improved, so did David's assignments. Rather than continue as a nightmare, school became more and more encouraging—for both David and his parents, and their relationship together.

Signs of an Eye-Hand Coordination Problem:

As a parent, any of the following signs might lead you to suspect that your child is experiencing difficulty with eye-hand coordination:

1. Your child has difficulty with spacing his words and keeping them on the line when writing.

2. Your child's handwriting is poor.

3. Your child does not seem to use his eyes to guide his hands to stay inside the lines when coloring. He avoids coloring, drawing, or maze-tracing activities.

4. When working with written math problems, your child has difficulty keeping the columns lined up.

5. Your child easily understands and can discuss what he has heard but has difficulty getting his thoughts down on paper.

Summary

The visual ability of eye-hand coordination is important whenever your child has to "get things down on paper." Difficulty in this area can cause extreme frustration in subjects in which writing is required. If your child demonstrates any of the behaviors described in this chapter, a complete vision evaluation which includes testing in the area of eye-hand coordination is indicated.

CHAPTER 11

"This Child Will Never Learn to Spell!"

Michael's Story

Michael was twelve years old. For some years in school he had experienced difficulty learning to sound out words. In first grade not only had he failed to remember which sound went with which letter, he frequently would not recognize a word that he had "learned" in the previous line. Repeating first grade did not solve the problem. Michael continued to struggle.

As the school recognized that Michael's difficulty was not based on "maturity," he began to receive special classes in reading. Despite these efforts, he continued to fall further behind.

In addition to having trouble with reading, Michael did not seem to be able to spell. Instead of spelling words correctly, he continued to spell them as they sounded. For example, Michael was likely to spell the word "enough" as "enuf," and the word "nation" as "nashun." As a result, Michael and his parents had been told by an "expert" that he "would never learn how to spell."

When I examined Michael, I found that he, like most of the children we see, was having difficulty with several visual abilities. One such ability was *eye teaming*.

As we discussed in Chapter 7, children with eye teaming problems either see the words run together or prematurely fatigue when struggling to keep the words single. This struggle was one of the reasons why Michael was not benefiting as he should have from his special help in school. After we had developed Michael's eye teaming ability, his reading was smoother, he made fewer careless errors, and he could read for longer periods of time without fatiguing. As a result, he was now able to respond to his school reading program.

Despite his improvement, however, Michael still had some problems picturing in his mind what he was reading about, and he definitely could not spell!

At this point we began to work with Michael's *visual imagery* ability. Visual imagery is the ability to "see the pictures" in your mind. For our purposes, this ability can be divided into two separate catagories: 1) the ability to retrieve or remember a picture of what has been seen in the past, and 2) the ability to create new pictures to view in your mind.

Visual Memory

The ability to retrieve or remember a picture in the mind that has been seen in the past is called *visual memory*. Being able to picture in your mind something you saw when you were last at the store would be one example of visual memory. Being able to picture in your mind where you left your car keys would be another example. A third example of visual memory would be the ability to see a picture in your mind of a word that you had seen in the past. For instance, look at the following word:

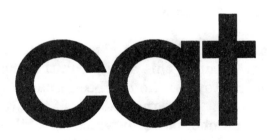

Now close your eyes and try to see a picture of the word. Open your eyes and look at the word again then close your eyes and repeat trying to see the word in your mind. Repeat this process several times until you can see the word "CAT" in your mind.

When performing this exercise, you may have a very clear picture of the word "CAT," or you may have only a vague impression of what was seen, like a half-remembered dream from the past. The picture may be straight ahead, or it may be hard to find, almost lost off to the side.

Even some very intelligent adults have difficulty with visual memory. If your own visual memory ability is undeveloped, you may be totally unable to recall any picture at all.

While there are good spellers who do not have good visual memory, good visual memory can be a real asset to spelling. The child who merely has to picture a word in his mind and then write down what he is seeing has a real advantage over the child who has to try to spell each word "as it sounds."

Because it is frequently possible to develop a child's visual memory, this ability can then be used by the child to spell even if he has been unable to master phonics or cannot "hear" the spelling of the word in his mind. As the number of words which the child can spell increases, the ability to recognize those words when reading also increases. In this manner, even the child who has had persistent problems with sounding out words can now use visual memory to work around that problem.

Visualization

The ability to form new pictures in your mind is called *visualization*. One example of visualization would be to picture in your mind how your living room would look if you rearranged the furniture. This same form of visualization could be used by the math student to picture the next step of a math problem before actually performing the work with a pencil.

Another example of visualization would be to picture in your mind what you are reading about. For instance, if a child were reading a story about Africa in which a lion were chasing a zebra the child would be better able to understand and remember the story if he could form a picture in his mind of the lion and zebra. The ability to picture, and, therefore, understand and remember what is read, is not only useful for reading books about Africa. This ability can also aid your child to get the most out of what is read, be it reading schoolwork or the word of God.

In Michael's case, as we worked on his visual memory and visualization skills, his ability to picture and remember what he was reading improved. Possibly even more exciting to Michael, however, was another newly developed ability: he could now picture words in his mind and accurately write those words down on paper. Not bad, for a child who "would never learn to spell!"

Signs of Difficulty with Visual Imagery Ability

1. Your child has persistent difficulty learning to spell.

2. Your child fails to recognize the same word in the next line.

3. Your child fails to "picture in his mind" what is read.

4. Your child has difficulty recalling what he did during the day or what he saw on the way home from school.

5. When your child loses his place during reading or boardwork he has difficulty remembering where he was so that he can find his place.

Summary

Visual imagery is the ability to "see pictures in the mind." There are two types of visual imagery. We call the ability to remember images from the past *visual memory*. We call the ability to form new images *visualization*.

These two abilities are important tools which, in many cases, can be developed with proper intervention. The child with poor visual imagery has to struggle that much harder to spell and read. The child with good visual imagery can not only recall the past, he can plan for the future.

A visual evaluation which goes beyond checking for 20/20 eyesight is the first step in determining the extent to which imagery ability is directing your child's success or failure in school—and life.

SECTION 3
Finding Help

CHAPTER 12

Ending the Struggle

A s we have discussed in the "Beyond 20/20" section of this book (Chapters 5 through 11), the *visual abilities* are the skills which give your child the power or means to take in information through his eyes.

Children who possess these abilities have the visual tools they need to perform at school. Children who lack these abilities have to struggle to make their way. For some, the struggle may allow them to get by but not reach their potential. For others the struggle is too great. They fail—usually without understanding why.

In the past chapters, as you read the children's stories, you may have "seen" your own child described and wondered "What can be done to help?" Chapter 12 is designed to answer this question. After briefly re viewing the visual abilities, we will discuss how they may be improved.

The Seven Visual Abilities for Learning

Although there are other visual abilities, the following are the main ones which affect learning.

20/20 ACUITY (Chapter 2)

20/20 Acuity is the ability to TEMPORARILY see tiny letters at twenty feet. Without this ability, your child will likely struggle to see the chalkboard in school. If your child lacks 20/20 acuity, it is likely that glasses will be prescribed.

Of the seven visual abilities necessary for school success, 20/20 acuity is the best known. Both school vision screenings and routine eye examinations check for this ability. Unfortunately, acuity is the only ability for which most screenings and routine exams do check.

ACCOMMODATION (FOCUS) ABILITY (Chapter 6)

Accommodation is the ability to MAINTAIN clear vision at all distances. Thus even the child with 20/20 vision, needs good accommodation ability to see clearly at reading distance or when shifting attention from chalkboard to paper.

EYE TEAMING ABILITY (Chapter 7)

Eye Teaming is the ability to coordinate the two

eyes together so that they both point at precisely the same object. If your child has deficient eye teaming ability, he may see double.

Of all the visual abilities, *Accommodation* and *Eye Teaming* are the two which are most crucial for good reading. Without these abilities, your child is likely to suffer from premature fatigue and loss of comprehension as he struggles to keep the print clear and single. These two abilities are needed for readers of ALL ages.

EYE MOVEMENT ABILITY (Chapter 8)

Eye Movement Ability includes moving the eyes from point to point (such as required in reading), following a moving object with the eyes (such as required for catching a ball), or holding the eyes stationary (such as required for maintaining eye contact during a conversation).

If your child lacks Eye Movement Ability, he is likely to lose his place when reading and make seemingly careless errors.

VISUAL PERCEPTION ABILITY (Chapter 9)

Visual Perception Ability is the ability to compare and understand things which are seen. Your child needs this basic skill to recognize letters or words when learning to read.

EYE-HAND COORDINATION ABILITY (Chapter 10)

Eye-Hand Coordination is the ability to use the eyes to guide the hands. Your child needs this skill to write neatly, align columns in math, complete board-work on time, or get his thoughts down on paper.

VISUAL IMAGERY ABILITY (Chapter 11)

Visual Imagery is the ability to remember or form pictures in the mind. If this skill is developed and used, your child will be able to "see" his spelling words in his mind and also picture in his mind what he is reading.

"Eyesight" versus "Vision"

When we use the word *eyesight* we are referring to *Visual Acuity*. Eyesight is the first of the seven visual abilities described above. Routine eye examinations check for eyesight.

When doctors say that your child's "eyes" are "fine" they are generally referring to eyesight. They mean that your child's eyes are healthy, that your child has 20/20 vision, and that your child does not need glasses to compensate for *nearsightedness, farsightedness,* or *astigmatism* (see Chapter 4). If your child does have a problem with eyesight, the doctor will generally prescribe glasses.

When we use the term *vision* we are not just referring to your child's eyes. We are referring to how your child USES those eyes to communicate with the world. In other words, *vision* is made up of all seven of the described visual abilities—and more!

If your child has perfect eyesight, he can see tiny letters at twenty feet for as long as it takes to read the acuity chart.

If your child has perfect *vision,* he can comfortably, continuously and effortlessly see at all distances (including reading distance) without any blurring or doubling. He can accurately aim his eyes (and his attention) at anything he chooses to inspect. He can easily see how details are similar or different and use his eyes to direct his hands or other body motions. He can remember what he has seen in the past and picture what he would like to accomplish in the future.

In addition to the above visual abilities, which are necessary for school, the child with good *vision* has additional abilities which prepare him for sports. He can tell how far away a ball is (*depth perception*) and see his teammates and opponents to the sides even when his eyes are directed straight ahead (*peripheral vision*). Children with good *vision* are seldom ridiculed by their teammates or left sitting on the bench.

The child with good *eyesight* does not need glasses to see the chalkboard. The child with good *vision* has the abilities he needs to perform at potential in life.

Vision is Learned

Vision, like other abilities is learned. While rarely

a child may come into the world with "faulty eyeballs" which require glasses or even surgery, that child's ability to use those eyes is learned.

For instance, sometimes a child will be born with one eye normal and the other eye farsighted. The child may then spend the first five years of his life with the condition left uncorrected. When, in kindergarten, the child's vision is finally screened and a referral to the eye doctor reveals the cause of the problem, glasses will be prescribed to compensate for the farsightedness in the one eye. Unfortunately, in many cases, the child may still be unable to see out of the farsighted eye even when wearing the glasses. The reason? Vision is learned!

During the years that the child's farsighted eye was left unfocused this learning did not occur. As a result, this child now has *amblyopia*. Amblyopia is a condition in which acuity is worse than 20/20 in one eye even though the eye is healthy and the "best" pair of glasses are being worn. For years, doctors believed that because "learning to see" out of an eye usually occurs before age six, it was useless to treat amblyopia after this age.

Actually, however, the belief that amblyopia cannot be treated after age six is a myth. Doctors Birnbaum, Koslowe, and Sanet—three faculty members at the State University of New York College of Optometry—reviewed EVERY published study on amblyopia treatment and found that both children and adults had a good chance of learning to read four lines further down the eye chart.

(See reference 14 in Appendix B.)

For example, if a patient began with 20/50 due to amblyopia, and as a result of treatment learned to see 20/40 then 20/30 then 20/25 and finally 20/20 he would have demonstrated four lines of improvement on the acuity chart. This improvement, Birnbaum, Koslowe and Sanet found, was as common AFTER AGE SIX-TEEN AS BEFORE AGE SIXTEEN. Based on this study, and hundreds of others, we now know that not only is vision learned, it can be taught—at any age!

This idea that vision is learned and can be taught at any age forms the basis for a form of treatment which has largely been developed within the vision-care profession of Optometry. The name of this form of treatment is *Vision Therapy*.

Vision Therapy is a process which relies on giving an individual feedback and practice to teach him to develop or enhance his visual abilities.

Vision Therapy is generally not a substitute for your child wearing the glasses needed to compensate for an eyesight problem. If your child has amblyopia, however, so that glasses do not fully improve acuity, then Vision Therapy can be used to improve this ability so your child can benefit from the glasses. Vision Therapy can also be used to teach your child the other visual abilities listed in this chapter.

As a result of Vision Therapy and the growing

number of specialists working in this area, many thousands of children across the nation no longer have to struggle because of deficient visual abilities. Words which used to run together no longer run together. Comprehension which used to reduce after a page of reading can now be maintained page after page. Children who used to complain about reading now read for fun. Handwriting which used to run up and down hill now stays on the lines. Spelling which used to consist of "kat" and "enuf" now appears as "cat" and "enough." Homework which used to take hours to complete is now finished to enjoy other pastimes. Constant frustration which used to consume both children and their parents is now reduced or even absent.

All of these changes are routinely occurring across the nation as the result of correctly applied Vision Therapy. Any of these changes may—depending on the results of a complete Vision Therapy evaluation—be available to your child.

Summary

In this chapter we have reviewed the visual abilities. We have also learned that because these visual abilities are learned, they can be taught through a process known as Vision Therapy. As a result of Vision Therapy, it may now be possible to end your child's struggle.

In the next chapter, we will provide more information on how Vision Therapy works.

CHAPTER 13

How Vision Therapy Works

As defined in Chapter 12, *Vision Therapy* is a process during which your child is given feedback and practice which teaches him to develop or enhance his *visual abilities*. This feedback is needed because abilities such as *accommodation* and *eye teaming* are not normally under your child's voluntary control.

The Stereoscope

During Vision Therapy we use numerous instruments to give your child feedback concerning eye teaming. One such instrument is called the *stereoscope*. This instrument consists of three parts (Figure 1).

1. Two windows to look through—one for each eye.

2. A divider between the two windows which separates the views seen by each eye. In this way, one target can be exposed to the right eye while a different target can be exposed to the left eye.

3. A card holder upon which the targets to be viewed are placed.

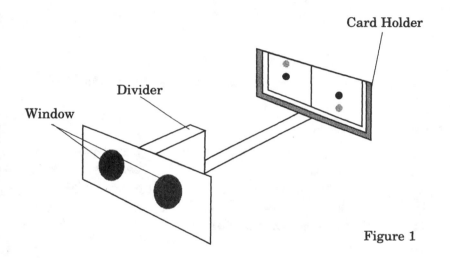

Card Holder

Divider

Window

Figure 1

In the stereoscope each eye sees its own target. The mind combines these two views into a single perception. For instance, if the left eye were shown a series of seven numbers and the right eye were shown an arrow, the mind would combine these two targets into a single perception of an arrow pointing at a series of numbers (Figure 2).

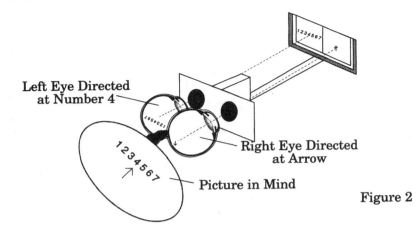

Left Eye Directed at Number 4

Right Eye Directed at Arrow

Picture in Mind

Figure 2

When the eyes were both aligned straight ahead, your child would see the arrow pointing at the number 4. If your child's eyes were pointing too far away he might see the arrow pointed at the number 2. If your child's eyes were pointing too close, he might see the arrow pointing at the number 6. In this manner, your child would have feedback when his eyes are aligned or not.

The Vision Therapy Sequence

While it is the instrument which gives a patient feedback, it is a skilled vision therapist who actually guides and coaches that patient toward improved visual abilities.

Although Vision Therapy is likely to vary somewhat depending on when and where an individual doctor was trained, the following is an example of the method we use at Cook Vision Therapy Centers. The example involves a child with an eye teaming problem.

1. Using the stereoscope described above, the therapist would first guide the child into understanding how the stereoscope works. The child would learn that when his eyes were accurately pointed at the target he would see the arrow pointed at the "number four." He would learn that when his eyes slipped too far outward the arrow would point to a lower number. Finally, he would learn that if he crossed his eyes too much, he would see the arrow pointing to a higher number.

2. Next, the therapist would "coach" the child to relax his eyes and "think about looking further away." As the child's eyes relaxed, he would see the arrow slide over toward the lower numbers. The therapist would then have the child "tighten" his eyes and "think about looking closer." The child would see the arrow move toward the higher numbers.

   Through practice and coaching the child would learn to align the arrow with any desired number.

3. Finally, the therapist would increase the difficulty of the task by having the child learn to effortlessly maintain the arrow pointed at the desired number four. As this procedure were practiced the child's

eye teaming ability would become more and more second nature.

In addition to using the stereoscope, the child would also work using many other instruments and procedures to develop his eye teaming. Each procedure would allow him to control his eyes with less effort. As a result of the variety of procedures used the child's improved eye teaming would be fully integrated into his way of seeing.

In this manner, the child would be *taught* to master the visual ability of eye teaming.

Summary

At Cook Vision Therapy Centers we use the three-step sequence described above with every Vision Therapy procedure and instrument. It does not matter if we are working with *20/20 acuity, accommodation, eye teaming, eye movements, visual perception, eye-hand coordination,* or *visual imagery*. Whatever the visual ability, the sequence is the same:

1. Your child is given feedback about some error in his vision system.

2. Your child is taught to control the error and know what he is doing that causes the error.

3. Your child then works with variations of the ther-

apy procedure until the new visual ability is integrated into his normal pattern of seeing.

Since incorporating this three-step sequence into our therapy programs, the length of those programs has reduced by almost 25 percent. Over 95 percent of the children who begin therapy go on to complete their programs and improve their visual abilities. Using this sequence it is possible to restore lost abilities or gain new abilities which allow the child better control of his vision, his schoolwork, and his life.

CHAPTER 14

Finding Help

I f you suspect that your child has difficulties with other than 20/20 ACUITY, where can you turn for help?

Although many eye doctors still center their exams around 20/20 acuity, an ever-increasing number of family *optometrists** are growing in their awareness of the importance to your child of the *visual abilities* which reach "beyond 20/20."

*An OPTOMETRIST is an eye doctor who diagnoses and treats both eye-health and vision problems as dictated by state law. In Georgia, for instance, optometrists are licensed to examine the health of the eyes, prescribe glasses and contact lenses, fit special devices for partially-sighted individuals, treat eye infections, and perform vision therapy. Optometrists from across the nation outnumber non-optometric eye care practitioners by two to one. While optometrists do not, as yet, perform eye surgeries, opthalmologists—the eye doctors who receive surgical but no optometric training—do not receive training in vision therapy for the majority of the visual abilities.

In 1980, when I first came to Atlanta to set up a practice specializing in *Vision Therapy*, only a handful of doctors were screening for and referring children with visual ability problems. Today, as the many studies (see Chapter 15) which support Vision Therapy have become known to those doctors who stay abreast in this area, we see patients referred by over 50 optometrists from across the state of Georgia.

Last year, optometrists from the Atlanta area alone attended over 300 hours of continuing education on the subject of Vision Therapy. The many family optometrists who are interested in keeping current on solving all of their patients' visual needs continue to expand their knowledge about referring patients for speciality care in Vision Therapy.

If your child's eye doctor is one who still does not ask specific questions about performance in reading and other schoolwork or does not seem to be helping you to solve these areas, there are organizations who can supply you with more information about Vision Therapy or—even better—help you to locate a specialist in Vision Therapy.

For more information about Vision Therapy you can write the Optometric Extention Program Foundation (OEPF). Founded in 1928, this organization is dedicated to education and research in VISION. The OEPF has a wealth of information designed to help parents understand vision and Vision Therapy.

The address for the OEPF is as following:

Optometric Extension Program Foundation (OEPF)
1921 East Carnegie Avenue, Suite 3L
Santa Ana, CA 92705

A second source of information regarding children's vision and Vision Therapy is the American Optometric Association (AOA). The AOA has well over 20,000 members from across the nation. This organization was founded in 1898. To obtain information from the AOA write the following address:

American Optometric Association
Communications Division
243 North Lindbergh Blvd.
St. Louis, MO 63141

All optometrists receive at least a basic introduction to Vision Therapy while working toward their Doctor of Optometry (O.D.) degrees. Those who go on to specialize in Vision Therapy, however, generally do so through additional training after completing optometry school.

To obtain the name of a specialist in Vision Therapy, write to the College of Optometrists in Vision Development (COVD). This organization certifies practitioners in the area of Vision Therapy.

To receive this certification and become a Fellow of COVD, an optometrist must wait three years after graduating from optometry school. This is to allow the practitioner time to develop adequate experience and training in Vision Therapy.

After the three-year period, the fellow-candidate must complete a process which includes passing a preliminary written exam, and submitting write-ups of Vision Therapy patients with whom the doctor has worked. When these requirements have been met, the doctor must pass both another written examination and an oral examination administered by the National Examination Board of COVD.

When this process is completed, the doctor becomes a Fellow in COVD (the initials for this distinction being F.C.O.V.D.). The doctor is then responsible for completing 30 hours a year of continuing education in order to continue to update his or her Vision Therapy skills.

To obtain the name of the nearest COVD Fellow, write the following address:

College of Optometrists in Vision Development
243 North Lindbergh Boulevard, Suite 310
St. Louis, MO 63141

Summary

If your child is struggling, frustrated, or performing below potential and your family eye doctor has not mentioned Vision Therapy as a possibility to look into, write for the name of a doctor who specializes in Vision Therapy. Then have your child receive a full evaluation to determine if there are deficient visual abilities which, if improved, might help reduce or end your child's struggle.

CHAPTER 15

Changing Children's Lives

Can you remember a time when someone helped you to do better? Taught you to ride a bike, perhaps? Showed you how to read or sew or play ball? Well, if you have experienced such help, then you know that in some areas at least, it is possible to be helped to learn a new skill and get better.

But can Vision Therapy help your child to do better? Turn to page 163 for a moment and then return to this page.

What you saw on page 163 was just a handful of the hundreds of research articles which support the effectiveness of Vision Therapy in producing desired results. The articles support the use of therapy for developing all of the *visual abilities* described in the ear lier chapters of this book.

If you have a background in the sciences and would like to examine the research for yourself, the majority of these articles (not to mention hundreds of others) are available through the following institution:

International Library, Archives & Museum of Optometry (ILAMO)
c/o American Optometric Association
243 N. Lindbergh Blvd.
St. Louis, MO 63141

Phone: (314) 991-0324

What Parents Say About Vision Therapy

Having been a faculty member at the State University of New York, having published in professional journals, and having helped to write the examination for the National Board of Examiners in Optometry (the organization which tests graduating optometry students for 49 of the 50 states), I am well aware of the importance of research in evaluating Vision Therapy.

In working with thousands of children over the past decade and a half, however, I am even more interested in what parents, such as yourself, have to tell me about changes seen in their children's lives.

The following comments are a sample of the many

hundreds accumulated over the past several years. These stories were written by the parents of children worked with at Cook Vision Therapy Centers. I believe they speak for themselves.

Jamie—Reason seen: Visual Perception, Eye Movements, Accommodation, Eye Teaming.

When Jamie started vision therapy she wrote her name backwards and really couldn't grasp the concept than an A was an A and never changes. Four months after starting...Jamie is in the 99% in visual discrimination [a form of visual perception] testing. And her self-esteem has increased enormously.

Thanks,

—TB

Joshua—Reason Seen: Eye-hand Coordination, Accommodation, Eye Movements, Eye Teaming.

Joshua (5 years old) was having a terrible time in school—hated it. The teacher said he had ADD [attention deficit disorder]. We brought him to Dr. Cook who found he had a vision problem with up-close work. He now loves school, likes to do table work (which he refused earlier) and has just calmed down some though he still has lots of energy.

Thank you Dr. Cook and staff for all the great help.

—DB

Charlie—Reason seen: Accommodation, Eye Teaming, Eye-hand Coordination.

Charlie started therapy in late November 1990. His goal was to be able to put distance between words and numbers. His work at school was sloppy and hard to read. After three visits I was surprised to see how nice Charlie was writing. His work was neat and his words didn't run together. Math was real interesting too...you could even tell one problem from another where before his math problems looked like a mess. Charlie's attitude changed too. After Christmas the school called to see if Charlie was on medication, his attitude was better and his work was so neat.

I feel vision therapy has truly helped Charlie with his schoolwork and attitude.

—MF

TINA—Reason seen: Eye Teaming, Accommodation.

She is able to read again. She would cry and get upset because when she read the words would double up and become blurry. She's always been one who read all the time. Thanks to Dr. Cook and vision therapy she can read till her heart's desire. Her headaches have also disappeared. Thanks from Tina and her parents.

—DH

Christopher—Reason seen: Eye Teaming, Accommodation, Eye Movements, Visual Imagery.

Christopher is more outgoing. His attention span is longer. His teacher says he is an excellent student. (last year he was "labeled" lazy!) He is doing very well in math and his first spelling test was 100. Last year he wasn't good in either of these areas. He now LIKES to read and even more important, he's not afraid to try new words.

Before he started vision therapy, school work was a source of frustration for Chris. Now he seems more able to deal with it on a daily basis.

—PT

Sarah—Reason seen: Accommodation, Eye Teaming

Before Sarah's vision screening was done at school, we knew there was a problem, but we didn't know what it was. She had such difficulty doing her school work and reading. When we told her we thought the problem had to do with her eyes and that we could fix it—it was like a huge weight lifted from her. Her self-esteem has risen. She is now reading independently. She completes her schoolwork on time. Sarah's teacher says she is almost like a different child. The improvement has been so dramatic. Both my husband and I are avid readers, so to have Sarah able to join us in this is too wonderful for words. Thank you all so very much.

—LR

Brian—Reason seen: Accommodation, Eye Teaming, Eye-hand Coordination.

Brian's ability to finish his work has improved greatly this year in school. His grades have improved, as has his self-esteem.

We have even noticed a change in his athletic ability. He is now able to hit a baseball!

Brain's handwriting in the third grade was not legible and now it is very neat.

—LD

Torrie—Reason Seen: Eye-hand Coordination, Accommodation, Eye Teaming, Visual Imagery.

Torrie's progress has been dramatic! She came in barely able to put letters on a straight line and now has such control over her handwriting that it looks as if it were professionally printed! She also has no more head-aches or hand cramps. Her math scores have also risen sharply—and she is able to complete her assignments in half the time. She is even beginning to do some recreational reading on her own. All of these changes have led to her feeling much more confident about her abilities—to the point that she told her teacher she "loved school." She entered vision therapy a pretty demoralized little girl, feeling that there was "something wrong with her." She is now back to her old out-going self. It has been like night and day!

We had really run the gamut of specialists from learning specialists to doctors of every sort. I came here wanting to be hopeful, but feeling very skeptical. I am convinced—and very grateful.

—LP

Conclusion

When entering optometry school in 1974, I had little notion of what the future would bring. As we studied the basic sciences and eye health and glasses and contact lenses, I was interested, but not yet enthusiastic, about the profession.

Then, in the third year we had a professor named William Ludlam. Dr. Ludlam had been involved in research at the Optometric Center of New York for many years before joining the faculty. While there, he completed three of the studies which are included in this book's Appendix on Research. In addition he had accumulated several decades of experience in private practice.

Somehow Dr. Ludlam was different than the other professors. He was not merely sharing information. He was excited. He taught one of the Vision Therapy courses. He told us stories of past patients' successes much like those contained inside this chapter. He shared the insights gained over years of study, research, and practical experience. He brought the subject alive.

During his many lectures, Dr. Ludlam would often repeat a phrase which somehow seemed out of place coming from a researcher and scientist: he told us again and again that in Vision Therapy we are "on the side of the angels."

Although, back then, I was somewhat cynical about such things, when Dr. Ludlam spoke he made it almost too real to disbelieve. Because of his influence, I specialized in Vision Therapy.

Now, fifteen years later, I look back at the many young faces we have seen pass from tears to smiles, the many lives we have changed, the many failures we have reversed, the many frustrations and struggles we have helped children conquer and I am amazed. On almost a daily basis we receive parents' comments, such as those reprinted in this chapter, and I wonder if Dr. Ludlam wasn't right.

But enough of the past. Let's look at the present. Let's look at the future. Is your child struggling? What effect does this struggle have on your child's life? What effect does it have on your life? What effect will it have five years from now?

If there is such a struggle, then it is time to end it. Use the information in this book to locate an optometrist who specializes in Vision Therapy. Call for an appointment.

Vision Therapy is not a "cure all." It only helps those who lack the visual abilities needed to succeed. If your child's examination reveals difficulties with visual abilities, then there is hope. There is help.

APPENDIX A
HELP FOR THE "CROSS-EYED" CHILD

In Chapter 7, we discussed *eye teaming* as the ability to point both eyes effortlessly and accurately at the same object. We mentioned that when the eyes slip, double vision is likely to occur.

"Crossed-eyes" is an extreme example of an eye teaming problem in which an eye slips in toward the nose. "Wall-eyes" is a similiar condition in which an eye drifts outward toward the ear. Eye doctors use the word *strabismus* to label these conditions. A child with strabismus has an eye which drifts in, out, up, or down. Sometimes both eyes drift.

The following story is about a child who had strabismus.

Hal's Story

Fifteen years ago I was called to the clinic to meet my first Vision Therapy patient. His name was Hal and he was nine years old. Hal was struggling in school and sports. He did not have the balancing ability to ride a bike. To make matters worse, his left eye was noticeably turned in toward his nose so his classmates made fun of him. Hal was not happy, and neither were his parents.

Talking to Hal's mother revealed that his left eye had been constantly turned in since he was a baby. For this reason, when I covered his right eye during his examination, he could not see clearly out of his left eye—either with or without glasses; having not used the eye while growing up, he had not learned to see out of that eye.

As described in Chapter 12, when acuity is worse than 20/20 in one eye even though that eye is healthy and the "best" pair of glasses are being worn, we call the condition *amblyopia*. Hal definitely had amblyopia. Having vision that could not be improved with glasses to better than 20/200, he could have been classified as being *legally blind* in his left eye.

In addition to not being able to see out of the left eye when the right eye was covered, Hal was unable to see out of the left eye when both eyes were open. As we explained in Chapter 7, when both eyes are accurately aimed at the object being viewed, the information coming from the two eyes will be combined in the mind in a single image (Figure 1). We call this combining or "melting together" of the images *fusion*.

If, however, one eye is aimed at the object being viewed and the other eye is turned to the side, the information from the two eyes will not be correctly combined in the mind and double vision will occur (Figure 2).

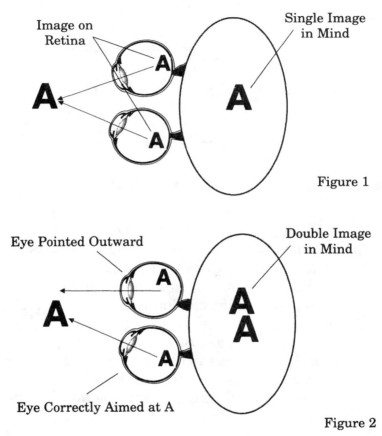

Figure 1

Figure 2

While the child with strabismus may at first see double, in time the mind will learn to ignore the extra image by ignoring all the information coming in through the turned eye. We call this ignoring the information entering one eye when both eyes are open *suppression* (Figure 3).

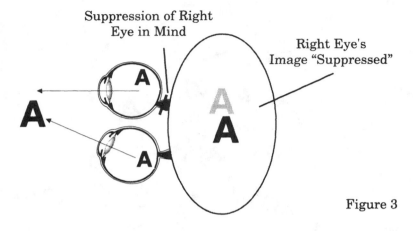

Figure 3

Suppression occurs at the expense of fusion. When the information from one eye is suppressed the mind is no longer combining information from the two eyes. Thus, the stronger suppression becomes the weaker fusion becomes. Since fusion is the "glue" which holds the two eyes in alignment, the less fusion there is the more the eye deviates. At the same time, the more the eye deviates, the less fusion there is. Thus, a "vicious cycle" occurs. In Hal's case, this "cycle" had gone on for so long that he had learned to completely suppress his left eye, and his eye was turned constantly.

Two-Eyed Depth Perception

Besides holding the eyes in alignment, the main advantage of fusion is improved depth perception.

The reason why depth perception is better when both eyes are used is that during two-eyed seeing each eye has a slightly different view of the same object. When these too different views are fused or melted together in the mind, the individual perceives a three-dimensional picture. This three-dimensional perception created by each eye having a slightly different view is called *stereopsis*.

The best way to understand stereopsis is to experience it. To do so, hold up two pens with one hand about ten inches in front of and half way between your eyes. Hold the pens with one about one inch to the side and about one inch in front of the other.

By covering one eye at a time with your free hand, look at the pens first with one eye and then with the other eye. Compare the two views to see how they differ. Then look with both eyes. Notice how much more space between the pens there appears to be with both eyes open. This perception of "extra space" is an example of stereopis.

Because stereopsis is dependant on fusion occuring, the more a child with strabismus suppresses his turned eye, the worse his stereopis will be. In Hal's case, he had no stereopsis whatsoever. This was the reason that such tasks as walking down stairs or riding a bicycle were difficult for him.

Treatment

When using Vision Therapy to treat a child with strabismus, we generally have two goals: 1) to improve how the child looks and 2) to improve how the child sees.

Children with strabismus are frequently concerned with their appearance. The younger child with strabismus may be called "cock-eyed" by other children on the playground. As the child grows older others may feel uncomfortable looking at him because it is difficult to tell which eye the child is using—the straight eye or the turned eye. These experiences can lead a child to avoid eye contact and, therefore, affect the child's relationships with others. For this reason, "how the child looks" is an obvious and major concern.

Unfortunately for children with strabismus, how the child "sees" is frequently overlooked. There are surgeries available, for instance, which can cosmetically straighten the child's eyes so that they "appear" straight. In the majority of cases, however, such surgeries do not, by themselves, eliminate suppression or establish fusion and stereopsis. Thus parents are given a false sense of security that the child "sees" better because he "looks" better.

Frequently, nothing could be further from the truth. Not only may these children continue to lack acceptable stereopsis, they may continue to demonstrate difficulties with such other *visual abilities* as *acuity*

(Chapter 2), *accommodation* (Chapter 6), *eye teaming* (Chapter 7) and any of the other visual abilities described in Chapters 8 through 11.

When we use Vision Therapy to teach a child to align his eyes, we improve the way the child "looks" by concentrating on how he "sees." As we improve the child's visual abilities such as accommodation, acuity, and eye teaming, his suppression is reduced and his fusion and stereopsis both improve. As fusion improves, the child begins to keep his eyes aligned for more and more of the day until "aligned eyes" becomes his normal way of seeing. More importantly, however, not only is he "looking" better, he is also "seeing" better and is, therefore, better prepared to succeed in school and life.

For some children with more noticeable eye-turns, a combined treatment which includes both surgery and Vision Therapy may be the best approach. With such a child, surgery would be used to grossly align the eyes, and Vision Therapy would be used to teach the child to use those eyes together. Since, as we stated earlier, fusion is the "glue" which holds the eyes in alignment, the child who receives Vision Therapy is less likely to require additional surgeries.

In Hal's case, he did not require surgery as part of his program. Because of the difficult nature of his problem, however, I worked with Hal for almost a year. At the end of that time, Hal's eyes were straight, his school and sports had improved, and he was now able to easily ride a bike. Hal, his parents, and myself were all delighted.

Summary

For the child with strabismus, Vision Therapy can ensure that his eyes actually work as a "team." If you have such a child and you wish to explore a non-surgical approach for helping your child, or if your child has already had surgery but you are still seeing that child struggle, make an appointment with an optometrist who specializes in Vision Therapy and find out what help is available.

APPENDIX B
Scientific Research:
50 Studies and Refereed
Articles About Vision Therapy

For the parents and patients who wrote the success stories "seeing is believing." But for those who feel more comfortable with research rather than anecdotal evidence, I'm including a list of 50 studies. You can find these articles at the International Library, Archives and Museum of Optometry (ILAMO). Phone 800-365-2219. E-mail ILAMO@aoa.org.

The articles support the use of vision therapy for improving eye-muscle coordination, depth perception, amblyopia (lazy eye) strabismus (crossed eyes) perceptual problems, and even visually-related reading problems. The Atzmon study, for instance, is a controlled medical study which shows the efficacy of vision therapy for reading difficulties associated with certain types of eye muscle coordination problems. About the study, Frimon E. Hardenbergh, M.D., Chief of Ophthalmology and Ophthalmologist to the Harvard University Health services wrote:

> "In my opinion, the prospective study was well planned and is essentially double blinded. . . The results support the proposition that application of orthoptics [a form of vision therapy] to all learning/reading disabled or deficient children who manifest convergence insufficiency [eye-teaming problems within arm's reach] should be the first line of therapy . . ."

The Studies

1) Atzmon, D., Nemet, P., Ishay, A., Karni, E.: A randomized prospective masked and matched comparative study of orthoptic treatment versus conventional reading tutoring treatment for reading disabilities in 62 children. *Binocular Vision and Eye Muscle Surgery Quarterly*, 1993, pages 91-106.

2) Birnbaum, M.H., Koslowe, K., Sanet, R.: Success in amblyopia therapy as a function of age. A literature review. *American Journal of Optometry and Physiological Optics*, 1977, pages 269-75.

3) Birnbaum, M.H., Soden, R., Cohen, A.H.: Efficacy of vision therapy for convergence insufficiency in an adult male population. *Journal of the American Optometric Association*, 1999, pages 225-232.

4) Buzzelli, A.R.: Stereopsis, accommodative and vergence facility: do they relate to dyslexia? *Optometry and Visual Science*, 1991, pages 842-846.

5) Ciufredda, K.J.: Goldrich S.G., Neary, C.: Use of eye movement auditory feedback in the control of nystagmus. *American Journal of Optometry and Physiological Optics*, 1982, pages 396-409.

6) Cohen, A.H., Soden, R.: Effectiveness of visual therapy for convergence insufficiencies for an adult population. *Journal of the American Optometric Association*, 1984, pages 491-494.

7) Cooper, J., Duckman, R.: Convergence insufficiency: Incidence, diagnosis and treatment. *Journal of the American Optometric Association*, 1978, pages 673-680.

8) Cooper, J., Feldman, J.: Operant Conditioning of fusional convergence ranges using random dot stereograms. *American Journal of Optometry and Physiological Optics*, 1980, pages 205-213.

9) Cooper, J., Selenow, A., Ciuffreda, K.J., et al.: Reduction of asthenopia in patients with convergence

insufficiency after fusional vergence training. *American Journal of Optometry and Physiological Optics,* 1983, pages 982-989.

10) Cooper, J., Medow, N.: Intermittent exotropia basic and divergence excess type. *Binocular Vision & Eye Muscle Surgery Quarterly*, 1993, pages 185-216.

11) Cornsweet, T.N.: Training the visual accommodative system. *Vision Research*, 1973, page 713-715.

12) Daum, K.: The course and effect of visual training on the vergence system. *American Journal of Optometry and Physiological Optics*, 1982, pages 223-227.

13) Daum, K.M.: A comparison of the results of tonic and phasic training on the vergence system. *American Journal of Optometry and Physiological Optics*, 1983, pages 769-775.

14) Daum, K.: Predicting results in the orthoptic treatment of accommodative dysfunction. *American Journal of Optometry and Physiological Optics*, 1984, pages 184-189.

15) Duckman, R.H.: Effectiveness of visual training on a population of cerbral palsied children. *Journal of the American Optometric Association*, 1980, pages 1013-1016.

16) Etting, G.: Strabismus therapy in private practice: cure rates after three months of therapy. *Journal of the American Optometric Association*, 1978, pages 1367-73.

17) Farrar, R., Call, M., Maples, W.C., A comparison of the visual symptoms between ADD/ADHD and normal children. *Optometry*, 2001, pages 441-451.

18) Flax, N., Duckman, R.H.: Orthoptic treatment of strabismus. *Journal of the American Optometric Association*, 1978, pages 1353-61.

19) Gallaway, M., Scheiman, M.: The efficacy of vision therapy for convergence excess. *Journal of the American Optometric Association,* 1997, pages 81-85.

20) Garzia, R., Richman, J.: Accommodative facility: a study of young adults. *Journal of the American Optometric Association*, 1982, pages 821-824.

21) Garzia, R.P.: The efficacy of visual training in amblyopia: A literature review. *American Journal of Optometry and Physiological Optics*, 1987, pages 393-404.

22) Goldrich, S.G.: Optometric therapy of divergence excess strabismus. *American Journal of Optometry and Physiological Optics*, 1980, pages 7-14.

23) Goldrich, S.G.: Oculomotor biofeedback and intermittent exotropia. *American Journal of Optometry and Physiological Optics*, 1982, pages 306-317.

24) Grisham, J.D., Bowman, M.C., Owyang, A., Chan, C.L.: Vergence orthoptics: validity and persistence of the training effect. *Optometry and Vision Science*, 1991, pages 441-451.

25) Halliwell, J.W., Solan, H.A.: The effects of a supplemental perceptual training program on reading achievement. *Exceptional Children*, 1972, pages 613-621.

26) Haynes, H.M., McWilliams, L.G.: Effects of training on near-far response time as measured by the distance rock test. *Journal of the American Optometric Association*, 1979, pages 715-718.

27) Hennessey D., Iosue, R.: Relation of symptoms to accommodative infacility of school-aged children. *American Journal of Optometry and Physiological Optics*, 1984, page 177.

28) Hoffman, L., Cohen, A.H.: Effectiveness of non strabismic optometric vision training in a private practice. *American Journal of Optometry and Archives of the American Academy of Optometry*, 1973, pages 813-816.

29) Hoffman L.H.: Incidence of vision difficulties in children with learning disabilities. *Journal of the American Optometric Association*, 1980, pages 447-451.

30) Hoffman, L.: The effect of accommodative deficiencies on the development level of perceptual skills. *American Journal of Optometry and Physiological Optics*, 1982, pages 254-262.

31) Hung, G.K., Ciuffreda, K.J., Semmlow, J.L.: Static vergence and accommodation: norms and orthoptic effects. *Documents of Ophthalmology*, 1986, pages 165-179.

32) Lieberman S.: The prevalence of visual disorders in a school for emotionally disturbed children. *Journal of the American Optometric Association*, 1985, pages 800-805.

33) Levine, S., Ciuffreda K.J., Selenow, A., et al.: Clinical assessment of accommodative facility in symptomatic and asymptomatic individuals. *Journal of the American Optometric Association*, 1985, pages 286-290.

34) Ludlam, W.M.: Orthoptic treatment of strabismus. *American Journal of Optometry and Archives of the American Academy of Optometry*, 1961, pages 369-388.

35) Ludlam, W.M., Kleinman, B.I.: The long range results of orthoptic treatment of strabismus. *American Journal of Optometry and Archives of the American Academy of Optometry*, 1965, pages 647-684.

36) Ludlam, W.M.: Visual training, the alpha activation cycle and reading. *Journal of the American Optometric Association.* 1979, pages 111-115.

37) Pavlidis, G.T.: Eye movements in dyslexia: Their diagnostic significance. *Journal of Learning Disabilities*, 1985, pages 42-50.

38) Poynter, H.L., Schor C., Haynes, H.M., et al: Oculomotor functions in reading disability. *American Journal of Optometry and Physiological Optics,* 1982, pages 116-27.

39) Press, L.J.: The interface between ophthalmology and optometric vision therapy. *Binocular Vision and Strabismus Quarterly*, 2002, pages 6-11.

40) Richman, J.E.: Use of a sustained visual attention task to determine children at risk for learning problems. *Journal of the American Optometric Association*, 1986, pages 20-26.

41) Saladin, J.J., Rick, J.O.: *Effect of orthoptic procedures on stereoscopic acuities. American Journal of Optometry and Physiological Optics*, 1982, pages 718-725.

42) Seiderman, A.S.: Optometric vision therapy—results of a demonstration project with a learning disabled population. *Journal of the American Optometric Association*, 1980, pages 489-493.

43) Sheedy, J.E., Saladin J.J.: Association of symptoms with measures of oculomotor deficiencies. *American Journal of Optometry and Physiological Optics*, 1978, pages 670-676.

44) Solan, H.A., Ficarra, A.P.: A study of perceptual and verbal skills of disabled readers in grades 4, 5, and 6. *Journal of the American Optometric Association*, 1990, pages 628-634.

45) Solan, H.A., Ficarra, A.P., Brannan, J.R., Rucker, F.: Eye movement efficiency in normal and reading disabled elementary school children: Effects of varying luminance and wavelength. *Journal of the American Optometric Association*, 1998, pages 455-464.

46) Solan, H.A., Larson, S., Shelley-Tremblay, J., et al.: Role of visual attention in cognitive control of oculomotor readiness in students with reading disabilities. *Journal of Learning Disabilities*, 2001, pages 107-118.

47) Suchoff, I.B., Petito, G.T.: The efficacy of visual therapy: Accommodative disorders and non-strabismic anomalies of binocular vision. *Journal of the American Optometric Association*, 1986, pages 119-125.

48) Vaegan, J.L.: Convergence and divergence show large and sustained improvement after short isometric exercise.

American Journal of Optometry and Physiological Optics, 1979, pages 23-33.

49) Wittenberg S., Brock F.W., Folsom, W.C.: Effect of training on stereoscopic acuity. *American Journal of Optometry and Archives of the American Academy of Optometry*, 1969, pages 645-653.

50) Zellers, J.A., Alpert, T.L. Rouse, M.W.: A review of the literature and a normative study of accommodative facility. *Journal of the American Optometric Association*, 1984, pages 31-37.

About the Author

Dr. David Cook (see www.cookvisiontherapy.com) limits his practice to vision therapy in metro Atlanta, Georgia. A former clinical instructor at the SUNY College of Optometry. He is the author of *VISUAL FITNESS: 7 Minutes to Better Eyesight and Beyond.* His professional articles have appeared in the top refereed optometric journals, and his "Eyesight, infinity and the human heart," was voted "Best Non-Technical Article by the Association of Optometric Editors in 1998.

Dr. Cook is a nationally known speaker on the topic of vision therapy. He has addressed the American Optometric Association, The American Academy of Optometry, the College of Optometrists in Vision Development, and the International Reading Association.

For five years, Dr. Cook served the National Board of Examiners in Optometry, co-chairing the committee which writes the questions on vision and learning. He also spent six years on the International Examination and Certification Board of the College of Optometrists in Vision Development, the group that board certifies optometrists in the area of vision therapy.

FOR ADULTS ONLY

VISUAL FITNESS QUIZ

Just as perfect hands don't guarantee the "hand fitness" to play piano, perfect eyes or new glasses don't guarantee the "visual fitness" to read *Harry Potter*, drive at night, or complete computer work without a headache. Which of the following statements apply to your life?

Reading
1. Reading puts you to sleep.
2. You lose concentration when reading.
3. Reading requires effort.

Driving
4. It worries you to drive after dark.
5. You get carsick.

Relationships
6. Headaches make you irritable.
7. You are too tired to enjoy your friends or family after a day of desk or computer work.

Sports and Coordination
8. In golf, you want to cut strokes.
9. In tennis, you want to sharpen your hand-eye reaction time.
10. In life, you want better coordination.

GETTING WORSE?

Visual Fitness

7 Minutes to Better Eyesight and Beyond

by Dr. David Cook

This book won't take the place of an eye exam. It's <u>not</u> about "throwing away your glasses." In fact, it's not about your eyes at all: *It's about how you use them!* It's your instruction manual for seeing smaller, longer, faster, for absorbing more information, for improving your eye-hand coordination and creating the *VISION* to change your world.

Visual Fitness
Buy It. Read It. Use It!

$13.00 – 222 pages – ISBN 0-425-19408-6

See a whole new difference in your sports, your energy level, your reading concentration and your relationships.

See a whole new difference In your outlook on life!
www.cookvisiontherapy.com